S272/05000778/31 ...
20 058
AF749067

A P... Eu... Gu... 2005

Northumbria University

Edited by

Peter Baskett FRCA, FRCP, FFAEM
Editor-in-Chief Resuscitation
Emeritus Consultant in Anaesthesia
Frenchay Hospital and Bristol Royal Infirmary
Bristol, UK

and

Jerry Nolan FRCA, FFAEM
Co-chairman International Liaison Committee on Resuscitation
Consultant in Anaesthesia and Intensive Care Medicine
Royal United Hospital
Combe Park
Bath, UK

WITHDRAWN

MOSBY
ELSEVIER

Edinburgh London New York Oxford Philadelphia St Louis Sydney Toronto 2006

MOSBY
ELSEVIER

© 2006 European Resuscitation Council. All rights reserved. Published by Elsevier Ltd.
First published 2006.

The rights of Peter Baskett and Jerry Nolan to be identified as the editors of this Work have been asserted by them in accordance with the Copyright, Designs and Patents Act 1988.

Front cover image © Will and Deni McIntyre/Science Photo Library, 327–329 Harrow Road, London W9 3RB, UK. www.sciencephotolibrary.com. All rights reserved.

No part of this publication may be reproduced, stored in a retrieval system, or transmitted in any form or by any means, electronic, mechanical, photocopying, recording or otherwise, without the prior permission of the Publishers or The European Resuscitation Council. Permission may be sought directly from Elsevier's Health Sciences Rights Department, 1600 John F Kennedy Boulevard, Suite 1800, Philadelphia, PA 19103-2899, USA: phone: (+1) 215 239 3804; fax (+1) 215 239 3805; or e-mail: healthpermissions@elsevier.com. You may also complete your request on-line via the Elsevier homepage (http://www.elsevier.com), by selecting 'Support and contact' and then 'Copyright and Permission'.

EAN: 9780723434238
ISBN: 0 7234 3423 9

British Library Cataloguing in Publication Data
A catalogue record for this book is available from the British Library

Library of Congress Cataloging in Publication Data
A catalog record for this book is available from the Library of Congress

Notice

Knowledge and best practice in this field are constantly changing. As new research and experience broaden our knowledge, changes in practice, treatment and drug therapy may become necessary or appropriate. Readers are advised to check the most current information provided (i) on procedures featured or (ii) by the manufacturer of each product to be administered, to verify the recommended dose or formula, the method and duration of administration, and contraindications. It is the responsibility of the practitioner, relying on their own experience and knowledge of the patient, to make diagnoses, to determine dosages and the best treatment for each individual patient, and to take all appropriate safety precautions. To the fullest extent of the law, neither the Publisher nor the Editors assumes any liability for any injury and/or damage to persons or property arising out or related to any use of the material contained in this book.

The Publisher

Working together to grow libraries in developing countries
www.elsevier.com | www.bookaid.org | www.sabre.org
ELSEVIER BOOK AID International Sabre Foundation

ELSEVIER your source for books, journals and multimedia in the health sciences
www.elsevierhealth.com

Printed in Spain.

The Publisher's policy is to use **paper manufactured from sustainable forests**

Contents

Preface

This pocket book contains the European Resuscitation Council Guidelines for Resuscitation 2005. It follows hard on the heels of the 2005 International Consensus Conference on Cardiopulmonary Resuscitation and Emergency Cardiovascular Care Science with Treatment Recommendations produced by the International Liaison Committee on Resuscitation published in *Resuscitation* in November 2005.

The European representatives at that conference, held in Dallas in January 2005, more than pulled their weight in the process of producing the Consensus on Science conclusions arising as a result of presentations and debate. Their names are listed at the end of this preface and the resuscitation community, in Europe and beyond, is most grateful to them for their talent, dedication and selfless hard work. In addition, they, and many others from Europe, also produced worksheets addressing the evidence for and against every conceivable detail of resuscitation theory and practice.

The European Resuscitation Council (ERC) Guidelines contain recommendations that, by consensus from the European representatives, are suitable for European practice in the light of today's conclusions agreed in the Consensus on Science. As with the Consensus on Science document, they represent an enormous amount of work by many people who have worked against the clock to produce the Guidelines for Europe. Each section of the guidelines has been masterminded and coordinated by the leaders of the ERC working groups and areas of special interest.

Such ventures do not happen without leadership and we are grateful to Vinay Nadkarni, Bill Montgomery, Peter Morley, Mary Fran Hazinski, Arno Zaritsky and Jerry Nolan for guiding the Consensus on Science process through to completion.

It would not be invidious to single out Jerry Nolan, the ILCOR Co-Chairman, for thanks and praise. He is universally respected and popular and has proved to be a wonderful ambassador for Europe. His scientific credibility and understanding is beyond doubt and his integrity, dedication, sheer hard work, patience and meticulous attention to detail and sensitivities have won the admiration of all. He has led the Consensus on Science process on our behalf and has been the lead coordinator in producing the European Guidelines. All this has been done unpaid in his own spare time and holidays and we are grateful to him, and to his family, for giving their all in these ventures. We are very lucky indeed to have such a man in our midst.

Finally we thank our Publishers, Elsevier, through the Publishing Editor for *Resuscitation*, Anne Lloyd, and her colleagues, for their professionalism, tolerance and patience in these ventures.

Representatives from Europe at the International Consensus Conference held in Dallas in January 2005

Hans-Richard Arntz (Germany), Dennis Azzopardi (UK), Jan Bahr (Germany), Dominique Bairent (Belgium), Gad Bar-Joseph (Israel), Peter Baskett (UK), Michael Baubin (Austria), Bob Bingham (UK), Bernd Böttiger (Germany), Leo Bossaert (Belgium), Steven Byrne (UK), Pierre Carli (France), Pascal Cassan (France), Sîan Davies (UK), Charles Deakin (UK), Burkhard Dirks (Germany), Volker Doerges (Germany), Hans Domanovits (Austria), Christoph Eich (Germany), Lars Ekstrom (Sweden), Peter Fenici (Italy), F Javier Garcia-Vega (Spain), Henrik Gervais (Germany), Anthony Handley (UK), Johan Herlitz (Sweden), Fulvio Kette (Italy), Rudolph Koster (Netherlands), Kristian Lexow (Norway), Perttu Lindsberg (Finland), Freddy Lippert (Denmark), Vit Marecek (Czech Republic), Koenraad Monsieurs (Belgium), Jerry Nolan (UK), Narcisco Perales (Spain), Gavin Perkins (UK), Sam Richmond (UK), Antonio Rodriquez Nunez (Spain), Sten Rubertsson (Sweden), Sebastian Russo (Germany), Jas Soar (UK), Eldar Soreide (Norway), Petter Steen (Norway),

Benjamin Stenson (UK), Kjetil Sunde (Norway), Caroline Telion (France), Andreas Thierbach (Germany), Christian Torp Pederson (Denmark), Volker Wenzel (Austria), Lars Wik (Norway), Benno Wolke (Germany), Jonathan Wyllie (UK), David Zideman (UK).

Peter Baskett and David Zideman

NORTHUMBRIA UNIVERSITY
LIBRARY
ITEM No. 200585834X
CLASS No 616.075 Poc

Chapter 1
Introduction

Jerry P Nolan

It is 5 y since publication of the Guidelines 2000 for Cardiopulmonary Resuscitation (CPR) and Emergency Cardiovascular Care (ECC). The European Resuscitation Council (ERC) based its own resuscitation guidelines on this document and these were published as a series of papers in 2001. Resuscitation science continues to advance and clinical guidelines must be updated regularly to reflect these developments and advise healthcare providers on best practice. In between major guideline updates (about every 5 y), interim advisory statements can inform the healthcare provider about new therapies that might influence outcome significantly.

The guidelines that follow do not define the only way that resuscitation should be achieved; they merely represent a widely accepted view of how resuscitation can be undertaken both safely and effectively. The publication of new and revised treatment recommendations does not imply that current clinical care is either unsafe or ineffective.

This pocket book version of the ERC Guidelines for Resuscitation 2005 contains all the key information that is presented in the full guidelines, but without the comprehensive reference list. This should enable resuscitation practitioners and trainers to gain access to all the relevant guidelines and algorithms conveniently and rapidly in a pocket book form.

Consensus on science

The International Liaison Committee on Resuscitation (ILCOR) was formed in 1993. Its mission is to identify and review international science and knowledge relevant to CPR, and to offer consensus on treatment recommendations. The process for the latest resuscitation guideline update began in 2003, when ILCOR representatives identified topics requiring evidence evaluation and appointed international experts to review them. To ensure a consistent and thorough approach, a worksheet template was created containing step-by-step directions to help the experts document their literature review, evaluate studies, determine levels of evidence and develop recommendations. A total of 281 experts completed 403 worksheets on 276 topics. Three hundred and eighty people from 18 countries attended the 2005 International Consensus Conference on ECC and CPR Science with Treatment Recommendations (C2005), which took place in Dallas in January 2005. Science statements and treatment recommendations were agreed by the conference participants and these were published as the 2005 International Consensus on Cardiopulmonary Resuscitation and Emergency Cardiovascular Care Science with Treatment Recommendations (CoSTR).

From science to guidelines

The resuscitation organisations forming ILCOR will publish individual resuscitation guidelines that are consistent with the science in the consensus document, but will also consider geographic, economic and system differences in practice, and the availability of medical devices and drugs. These 2005 ERC Resuscitation Guidelines are derived from the CoSTR document but represent consensus among members of the ERC Executive Committee. The ERC Executive Committee considers these new recommendations to be the most effective and easily learned interventions that can be supported by current knowledge, research and experience. Inevitably, even within Europe, differences in the availability of drugs, equipment and personnel will necessitate local, regional and national adaptation of these guidelines.

Demographics

Ischaemic heart disease is the leading cause of death in the world. Sudden cardiac arrest is responsible for more than 60% of adult deaths from coronary heart disease. Based on data from Scotland and from five cities in other parts of Europe, the annual incidence of resuscitation for out-of-hospital cardiopulmonary arrest of cardiac aetiology is 49.5–66 per 100,000 population. Data on the aetiology of out-of-hospital cardiac arrests is given in Table 1.1. The incidence of in-hospital cardiac arrest is difficult to assess because it is influenced heavily by factors such as the criteria for hospital admission and implementation of a do not attempt

Table 1.1 Out-of-hospital cardiopulmonary arrests by aetiology

	N (%) (n = 21,175)
Presumed cardiac disease	17,451 (82.4)
Non-cardiac internal aetiologies	1814 (8.6)
• Lung disease	901 (4.3)
• Cerebrovascular disease	457 (2.2)
• Cancer	190 (0.9)
• Gastrointestinal haemorrhage	71 (0.3)
• Obstetric/paediatric	50 (0.2)
• Pulmonary embolism	38 (0.2)
• Epilepsy	36 (0.2)
• Diabetes mellitus	30 (0.1)
• Renal disease	23 (0.1)
Non-cardiac external aetiologies	1910 (9.0)
• Trauma	657 (3.1)
• Asphyxia	465 (2.2)
• Drug overdose	411 (1.9)
• Drowning	105 (0.5)
• Electric shock/ lightning	28 (0.1)
• Other suicide	194 (0.9)
• Other external	50 (0.2)

Data from Pell JP et al. Heart 2003;89:839–42.

resuscitation (DNAR) policy. In a general hospital in the UK, the incidence of primary cardiac arrest (excluding those with DNAR and those arresting in the emergency department) was 3.3/1000 admissions; using the same exclusion criteria the incidence of cardiac arrest in a Norwegian University hospital was 1.5/1000 admissions.

The chain of survival

The actions linking the victim of sudden cardiac arrest with survival are called the chain of survival. The previous chain of survival included early recognition of the emergency and activation of the emergency services, early CPR, early defibrillation and early advanced life support. The infant and child chain of survival includes prevention of conditions leading to the cardiopulmonary arrest, early CPR, early activation of the emergency services and early advanced life support. In hospital, the importance of early recognition of the critically ill patient and activation of a medical emergency team (MET) is now well accepted. Previous resuscitation guidelines have provided relatively little information on treatment of the patient during the post-resuscitation care phase. There is substantial variability in the way comatose survivors of cardiac arrest are treated in the initial hours and first few days after return of spontaneous circulation (ROSC). Differences in treatment at this stage may account for some of the inter-hospital variability in outcome after cardiac arrest. The importance of recognising critical illness and/or angina and preventing cardiac arrest (in- or out-of-hospital), and post-resuscitation care has been highlighted by the inclusion of these elements in a new four-ring chain of survival (Figure 1.1). The first link indicates the importance of recognising those at risk of cardiac arrest and calling for help in the hope that early treatment can prevent arrest. The central links in this new chain depict the integration of CPR and defibrillation as the fundamental components of early resuscitation in an attempt to restore life. The final link, post-resuscitation care, is targeted at preserving function, particularly of the brain and heart.

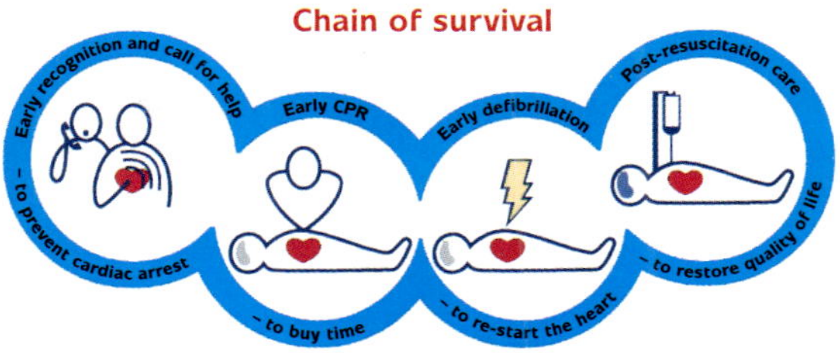

Figure 1.1. ERC chain of survival.

The universal algorithm

The adult and paediatric basic and advanced life support algorithms have been updated to reflect changes in the ERC guidelines. Every effort has been made to keep these algorithms simple, yet make them applicable to cardiac arrest victims in most circumstances. Rescuers begin CPR if the victim is unconscious or unresponsive, and not breathing normally (ignoring occasional gasps). A single compression–ventilation (CV) ratio of 30:2 is used for the single rescuer of an adult or child (excluding neonates) out of the hospital, and for all adult CPR. This single ratio is designed to simplify teaching, promote skill retention, increase the number of compressions given, and decrease interruption to compressions. Once a defibrillator is attached, if a shockable rhythm is confirmed, a single shock is delivered. Irrespective of the resultant rhythm, chest compressions and ventilations (2 min with a CV ratio of 30:2) are resumed immediately after the shock to minimise the 'no flow' time. Advanced life support interventions are outlined in a box at the centre of the algorithm. Once the airway is secured with a tracheal tube, laryngeal mask airway (LMA) or Combitube, the lungs are ventilated at a rate of 8–10 min^{-1} without pausing during chest compressions.

Quality of CPR

Interruptions to chest compressions must be minimised. On stopping chest compressions, the coronary flow decreases substantially – on resuming chest compressions it takes several compressions before the coronary flow recovers to its previous level. Recent evidence indicates that unnecessary interruptions to chest compressions occur frequently both in- and out-of-hospital. Resuscitation instructors must emphasise the importance of minimising interruptions to chest compressions.

Summary

It is intended that these new guidelines will improve the practice of resuscitation and, ultimately, the outcome from cardiac arrest. The universal ratio of 30 compressions to two ventilations should reduce interruptions in compression and the likelihood of hyperventilation, simplify instruction for teaching, and improve skill retention. The single shock strategy should minimise 'no flow' time.

Further reading

1. International Liaison Committee on Resuscitation. 2005 International Consensus on Cardiopulmonary Resuscitation and Emergency Cardiovascular Care Science with Treatment Recommendations. Resuscitation 2005;67:163–86.
2. European Resuscitation Council. European Resuscitation Council guidelines for resuscitation 2005. Resuscitation 2005;67(Suppl 1):S3–6.
3. Hodgetts TJ, Kenward G, Vlackonikolis I, et al. Incidence, location and reasons for avoidable in-hospital cardiac arrest in a district general hospital. Resuscitation 2002; 54:115–23.
4. Skogvoll E, Isern E, Sangolt GK, et al. In-hospital cardiopulmonary resuscitation. Five years incidence and survival according to the Utstein template. Acta Anaesthesiol Scand 1999;43:177–84.
5. Pell JP, Sirel JM, Marsden AK, et al. Presentation, management, and outcome of out of hospital cardiopulmonary arrest: comparison by underlying aetiology. Heart 2003;89:839–42.

Chapter 2 Adult basic life support and use of automated external defibrillators

Anthony Handley, Rudolph Koster, Koen Monsieurs, Gavin Perkins, Sîan Davies and Leo Bossaert

Basic life support (BLS) refers to maintaining airway patency and supporting breathing and the circulation without the use of equipment other than a protective device. This section contains the guidelines for lay rescuer adult BLS and for the use of an automated external defibrillator (AED). It also includes recognition of sudden cardiac arrest (SCA), the recovery position and management of choking (foreign body airway obstruction). Guidelines for in-hospital BLS and the use of manual defibrillators may be found in Chapters 3 and 4.

Introduction

Sudden cardiac arrest is a leading cause of death in Europe, affecting about 700,000 individuals a year. At the time of the first heart rhythm analysis, about 40% of SCA victims have ventricular fibrillation (VF). It is likely that many more victims have VF or rapid ventricular tachycardia (VT) at the time of collapse, but by the time the first ECG is recorded, their rhythm has deteriorated to asystole. The optimum treatment for VF cardiac arrest is immediate bystander CPR (combined chest compression and rescue breathing) plus electrical defibrillation. The predominant mechanism of cardiac arrest in victims of trauma, drug overdose, drowning and many children is asphyxia; rescue breaths are critical for resuscitation of these victims.

Victims of cardiac arrest need immediate CPR. This provides a small but critical blood flow to the heart and brain. It also increases the likelihood that a defibrillatory shock will terminate VF and enable the heart to resume an effective rhythm and effective systemic perfusion. Chest compression is especially important if a shock cannot be delivered sooner than 4 or 5 min after collapse. In the first few minutes after successful defibrillation, the rhythm may be slow and ineffective; chest compressions may be needed until adequate cardiac function returns.

Adult BLS sequence

Basic life support consists of the following sequence of actions (Figure 2.1):

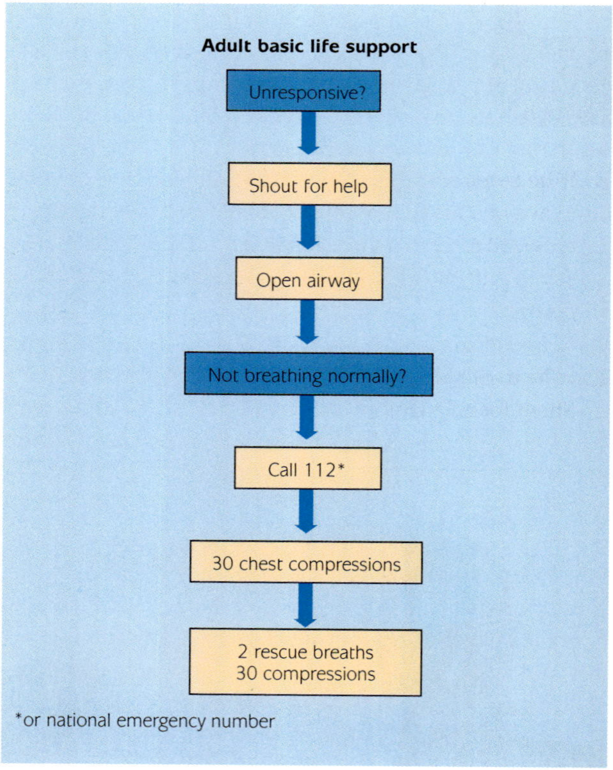

Figure 2.1. The BLS algorithm.

1. **Make sure you, the victim and any bystanders are safe.**
2. **Check the victim for a response** (Figure 2.2):

- Gently shake his shoulders and ask loudly: "Are you all right?"

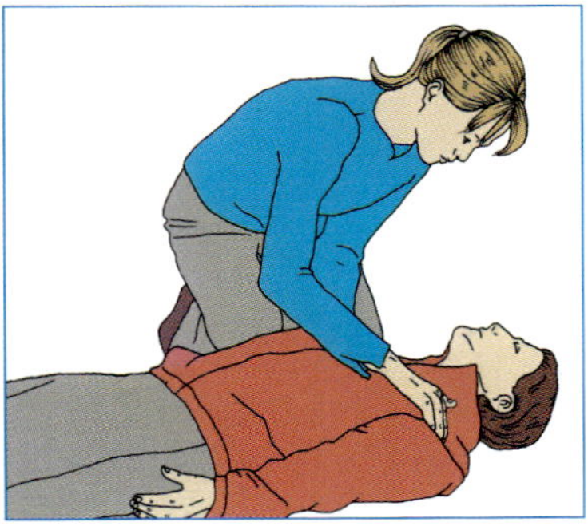

Figure 2.2. Check the victim for a response. © ERC 2005.

3A. If he responds:

- Leave him in the position in which you find him provided there is no further danger.
- Try to find out what is wrong with him and get help if needed.
- Reassess him regularly.

3B. If he does *not* respond:

- Shout for help (Figure 2.3).

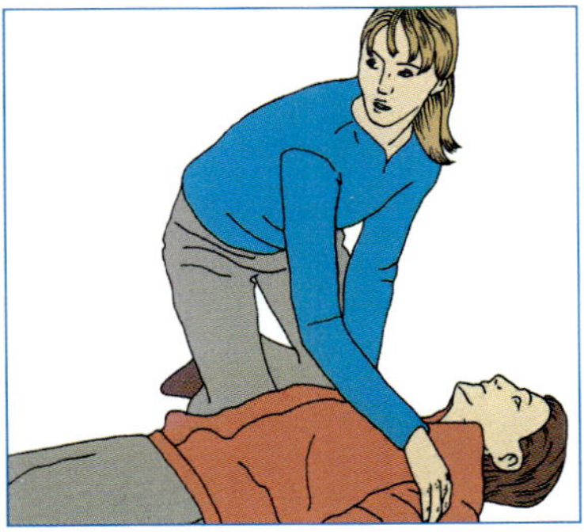

Figure 2.3. Shout for help. © ERC 2005.

- Turn the victim onto his back and then open the airway using head tilt and chin lift (Figure 2.4).

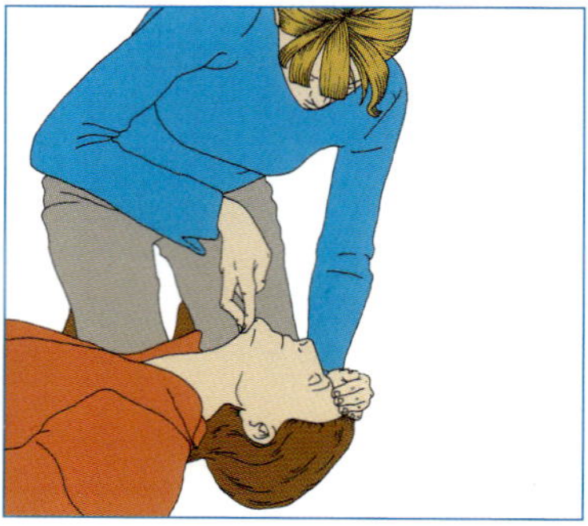

Figure 2.4. Place your hand on his forehead using head tilt and chin lift. © ERC 2005.

- Place your hand on his forehead and gently tilt his head back keeping your thumb and index finger free to close his nose if rescue breathing is required (Figure 2.5).
- With your fingertips under the point of the victim's chin, lift the chin to open the airway.

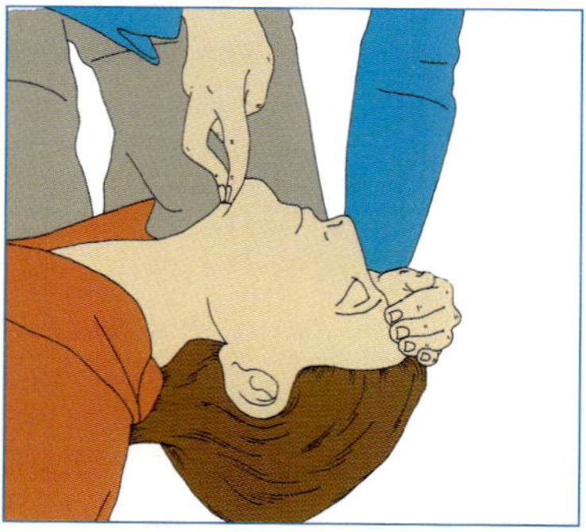

Figure 2.5. Gently tilt his head back. © ERC 2005.

4. **Keeping the airway open, look, listen and feel for normal breathing** (Figure 2.6):

- Look for chest movement.
- Listen at the victim's mouth for breath sounds.
- Feel for air on your cheek.

In the first few minutes after cardiac arrest, a victim may be barely breathing, or taking infrequent, noisy, gasps. Do not confuse this with normal breathing.

Look, listen and feel for *no more* than *10 s* to determine if the victim is breathing normally. If you have any doubt whether breathing is normal, act as if it is *not* normal.

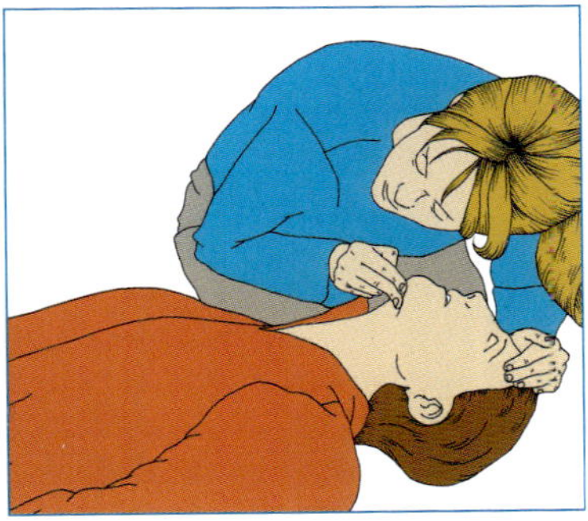

Figure 2.6. Look, listen and feel for normal breathing. © ERC 2005.

5A. If he *is* breathing normally:

- Turn him into the recovery position (see section below on 'Recovery position').
- Send or go for help/call for an ambulance.
- Check for continued breathing.

5B. If he is *not* breathing normally:

- Send someone for help or, if you are on your own, leave the victim and alert the ambulance service; return and start chest compression as follows:
  - Kneel by the side of the victim
  - Place the heel of one hand in the centre of the victim's chest (Figure 2.7)

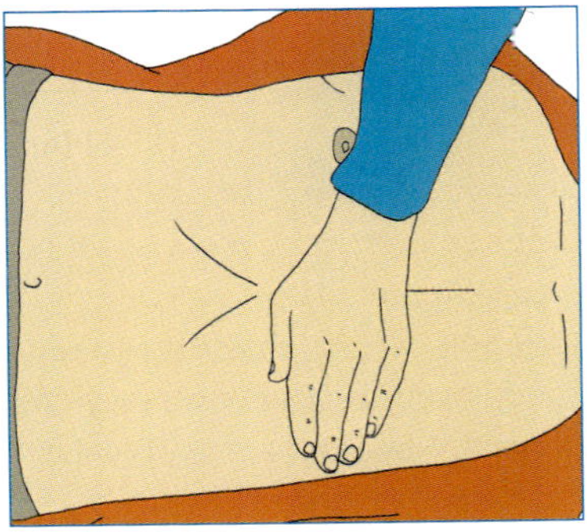

Figure 2.7. Place the heel of one hand in the centre of the chest. © ERC 2005.

- Place the heel of your other hand on top of the first hand (Figure 2.8).

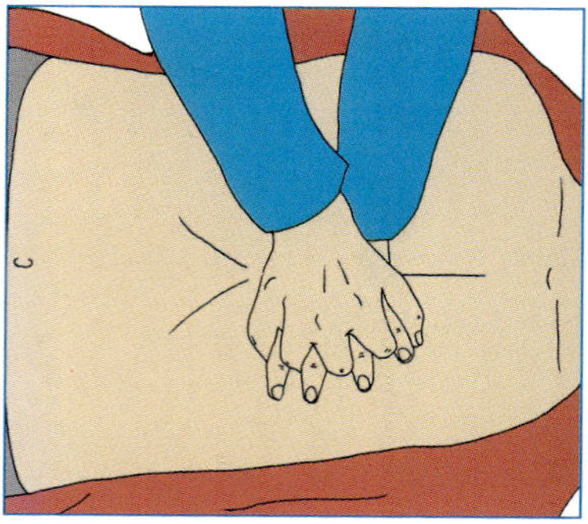

Figure 2.8. Place the heel of your other hand on top of the first hand. © ERC 2005.

- Interlock the fingers of your hands and ensure that pressure is not applied over the victim's ribs. Do not apply any pressure over the upper abdomen or the bottom end of the bony sternum (breastbone) (Figure 2.9).

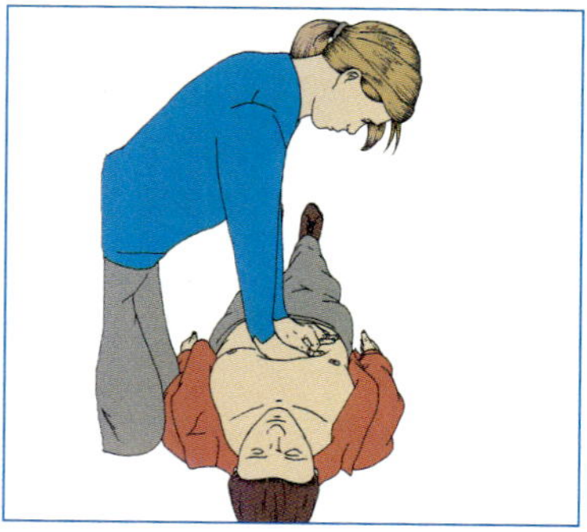

Figure 2.9. Interlock your fingers and apply pressure over the sternum. © ERC 2005.

- Position yourself vertically above the victim's chest and, with your arms straight, press down on the sternum 4–5 cm (Figure 2.10).
- After each compression, release all the pressure on the chest without losing contact between your hands and the sternum. Repeat at a rate of about

100 times a minute (a little less than two compressions a second).

- Compression and release should take an equal amount of time.

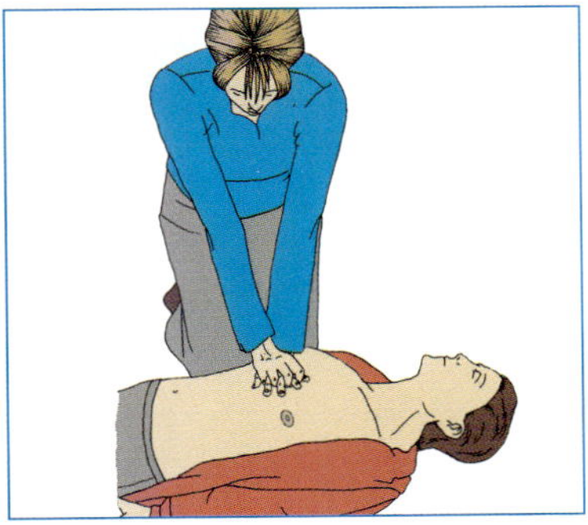

Figure 2.10. Compress the sternum 4–5 cm. © ERC 2005.

6A. Combine chest compression with rescue breaths:

- After 30 compressions, open the airway again using head tilt and chin lift (Figure 2.11).
- Pinch the soft part of his nose closed, using the index finger and thumb of your hand on his forehead.
- Allow his mouth to open, but maintain chin lift.
- Take a normal breath and place your lips around his mouth, making sure that you have a good seal.

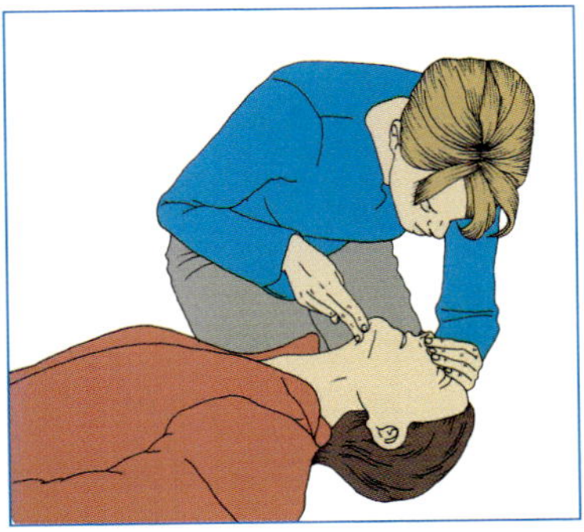

Figure 2.11. Open the airway. © ERC 2005.

- Blow steadily into his mouth whilst watching for his chest to rise; take about 1 s to make his chest rise as in normal breathing; this is an effective rescue breath (Figure 2.12).

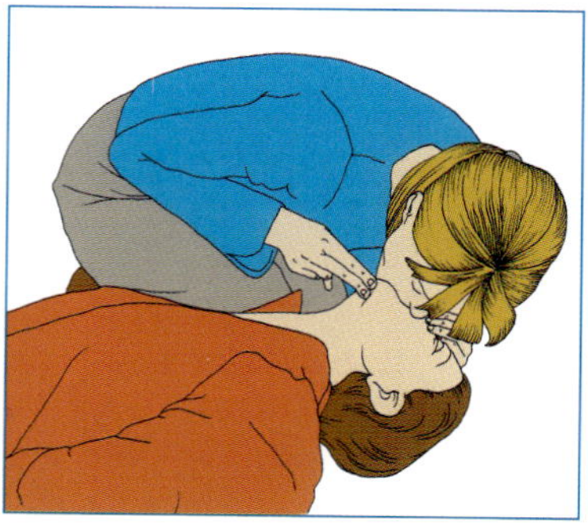

Figure 2.12. Blow steadily into his mouth watching for the chest to rise. © ERC 2005.

- Maintaining head tilt and chin lift, take your mouth away from the victim and watch for his chest to fall as air comes out (Figure 2.13).

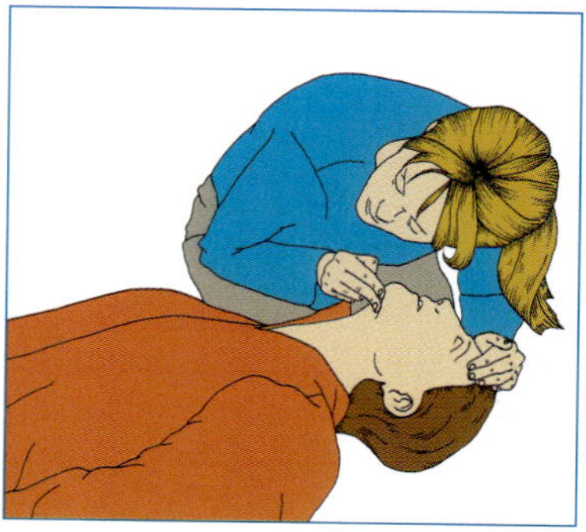

Figure 2.13. Take your mouth away and watch for the chest to fall. © ERC 2005.

- Take another normal breath and blow into the victim's mouth once more to give a total of two effective rescue breaths. Then return your hands without delay to the correct position on the sternum and give a further 30 chest compressions.
- Continue with chest compressions and rescue breaths in a ratio of 30:2.

- Stop to recheck the victim only if he starts breathing *normally*; otherwise *do not interrupt resuscitation.*

If your initial rescue breath does not make the chest rise as in normal breathing, then before your next attempt:

- Check the victim's mouth and remove any obstruction.
- Recheck that there is adequate head tilt and chin lift.
- Do not attempt more than two breaths each time before returning to chest compressions.

If there is more than one rescuer present, another should take over CPR every 1–2 min to prevent fatigue. Ensure the minimum of delay during the change-over of rescuers.

6B. Chest compression-only CPR:

- If you are not able or are unwilling to give rescue breaths, give chest compressions only.
- If chest compressions only are given, these should be continuous at a rate of 100 min^{-1}.
- Stop to recheck the victim only if he starts breathing *normally*; otherwise do not interrupt resuscitation.

7. Continue resuscitation until:

- Qualified help arrives and takes over.
- The victim starts breathing normally.
- You become exhausted.

Risk to the rescuer

The safety of both the rescuer and victim is paramount during a resuscitation attempt. There have been few incidents of rescuers suffering adverse effects from undertaking CPR, with only isolated reports of infections such as tuberculosis (TB) and severe acute respiratory distress syndrome (SARS). Transmission of HIV during CPR has never been reported. There have been no human studies to address the effectiveness of barrier devices during CPR; however, laboratory studies have shown that certain filters, or barrier devices with one-way valves, prevent oral bacteria transmission from the victim to the rescuer during mouth-to-mouth ventilation. Rescuers should take appropriate safety precautions where feasible, especially if the victim is known to have a serious infection, such as TB or SARS. During an outbreak of a highly infectious condition such as SARS, full protective precautions for the rescuer are essential.

Opening the airway

The jaw thrust is not recommended for lay rescuers because it is difficult to learn and perform and may itself cause spinal movement. Therefore, the lay rescuer should open the airway using a head tilt–chin lift manoeuvre for both injured and non-injured victims.

Recognition of cardiorespiratory arrest

Checking the carotid pulse is an inaccurate method of confirming the presence or absence of circulation. Healthcare professionals as well as lay rescuers have difficulty determining the presence or absence of adequate or normal breathing in unresponsive victims. This may be because the airway is not open or because the victim is making occasional (agonal) gasps. Agonal gasps are present in up to 40% of cardiac arrest victims. Lay people should be taught to begin CPR if the victim is unconscious (unresponsive) and not breathing normally. It should be emphasised during training that agonal gasps occur commonly in the first few minutes after SCA. They are an indication for starting CPR immediately and should not be confused with normal breathing.

Initial rescue breaths

It is well recognised that skill acquisition and retention is aided by simplification of the BLS sequence of actions. It is also recognised that rescuers are frequently unwilling to carry out mouth-to-mouth ventilation for a variety of reasons, including fear of infection and distaste for the procedure. For these reasons, and to emphasise the priority of chest compressions, it is recommended that, in adults, CPR should start with chest compression rather than initial ventilation.

Ventilation

During CPR, the purpose of ventilation is to maintain adequate oxygenation. The optimal tidal volume, respiratory rate and inspired oxygen concentration to achieve this, however, are not fully known. Based on the available science, the recommendation is for rescuers to give each rescue breath over about 1 s, with enough volume to make the victim's chest rise, but to avoid rapid or forceful breaths. This recommendation applies to all forms of ventilation during CPR, including mouth-to-mouth and bag-mask (BM) with and without supplementary oxygen.

Mouth-to-nose ventilation

Mouth-to-nose ventilation is an effective alternative to mouth-to-mouth ventilation. It may be considered if the victim's mouth is seriously injured or cannot be opened, the rescuer is assisting a victim in the water, or a mouth-to-mouth seal is difficult to achieve.

Mouth-to-tracheostomy ventilation

There is no published evidence on the safety, effectiveness or feasibility of mouth-to-tracheostomy ventilation, but it may be used for a victim with a tracheostomy tube or tracheal stoma who requires rescue breathing.

Bag-mask ventilation

To use bag-mask ventilation requires considerable practice and skill. It is a technique that is appropriate only for lay rescuers who work in highly specialised areas, such as where there is a risk of cyanide poisoning or exposure to other toxic agents.

Chest compression

Chest compressions generate a small but critical amount of blood flow to the brain and myocardium and increase the likelihood that defibrillation will be successful. They are especially important if the first shock is delivered more than 5 min after collapse.

The conclusions of the 2005 Consensus Conference included:

1. Each time compressions are resumed, the rescuer should place his hands without delay 'in the centre of the chest'.
2. The chest should be compressed at a rate of about 100 min^{-1}.
3. Attention should be paid to achieving the full compression depth of 4–5 cm (for an adult).
4. The chest should be allowed to recoil completely after each compression.
5. Approximately the same amount of time should be taken for compression as for relaxation.
6. Interruptions in chest compression should be minimised.
7. Palpation of the carotid or femoral pulse should not be used as a gauge of effective arterial flow.

Previous guidelines have recommended finding the middle of the lower half of the sternum by placing one finger on the lower end of the sternum and sliding the other hand down to it. It has been shown that for healthcare professionals the same hand position can be found more quickly if rescuers are taught to 'place the heel of your hand in the centre of the chest with the other hand on top', provided the teaching includes a demonstration of placing the hands in the middle of the lower half of the sternum. It is reasonable to extend this to lay people

'Compression rate' refers to the speed at which compressions are given, not the total number delivered in each minute. The number delivered is determined by the rate, but also by the number of interruptions to open the airway, deliver rescue breaths and allow AED analysis.

Compression–ventilation ratio

Insufficient evidence from human outcome studies exists to support any given compression:ventilation ratio. Animal data and a mathematical model suggest that a ratio of 30:2 should provide the best compromise between blood flow and oxygen delivery.

A ratio of 30 compressions to two ventilations is, therefore, recommended for the single rescuer attempting resuscitation on an adult or child out of hospital.

Compression-only CPR

Healthcare professionals as well as lay rescuers admit to being reluctant to perform mouth-to-mouth ventilation in unknown victims of cardiac arrest.

In adults, the outcome of chest compression without ventilation is significantly better than the outcome of giving no CPR. Lay people should, therefore, be encouraged to do compression-only CPR if they are unable or unwilling to provide rescue breaths, although combined chest compression and ventilation is the better method of CPR.

Recovery position

There are several variations of the recovery position, each with its own advantages. No single position is perfect for all victims. The position should be stable, near a true lateral position with the head dependent, and with no pressure on the chest to impair breathing.

The ERC recommends this sequence of actions to place a victim in the recovery position:

- Remove the victim's spectacles.
- Kneel beside the victim and make sure that both his legs are straight.
- Place the arm nearest to you out at right angles to his body, elbow bent with the hand palm uppermost (Figure 2.14).

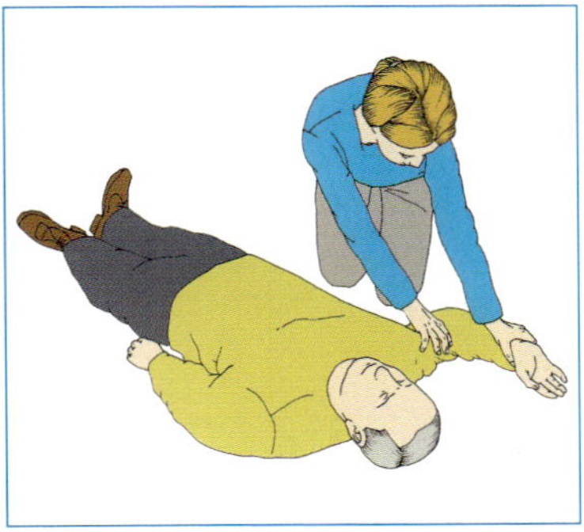

Figure 2.14. Place the arm nearest to you out at right angles to his body, elbow bent with the hand palm uppermost. © ERC 2005.

- Bring the far arm across the chest, and hold the back of the hand against the victim's cheek nearest to you (Figure 2.15).

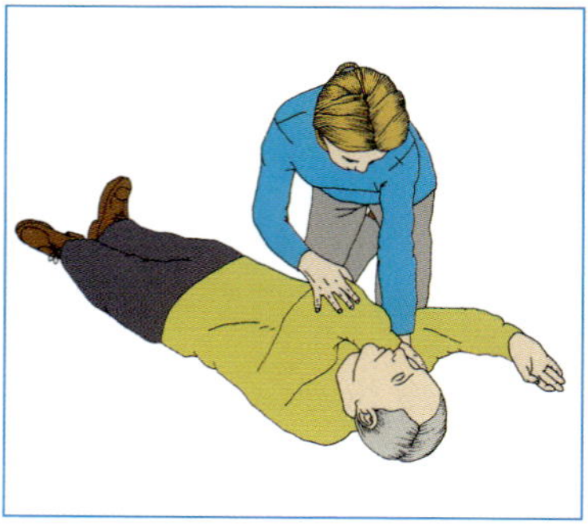

Figure 2.15. Bring the far arm across the chest, and hold the back of the hand against the victim's cheek nearest to you. © ERC 2005.

- With your other hand, grasp the far leg just above the knee and pull it up, keeping the foot on the ground (Figure 2.16).
- Keeping his hand pressed against his cheek, pull on the far leg to roll the victim towards you onto his side.
- Adjust the upper leg so that both the hip and knee are bent at right angles.
- Tilt the head back to make sure the airway remains open.

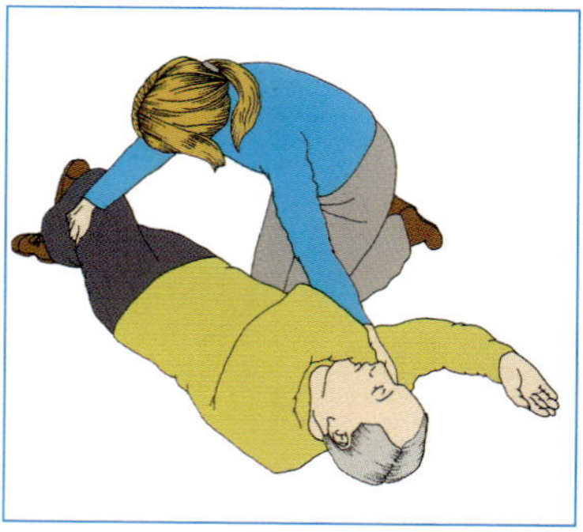

Figure 2.16. With your other hand, grasp the far leg just above the knee and pull it up, keeping the foot on the ground. © ERC 2005.

- Adjust the hand under the cheek, if necessary, to keep the head tilted (the recovery position) (Figure 2.17).
- Check breathing regularly.

If the victim has to be kept in the recovery position for *more than 30 min* turn him to the opposite side to relieve the pressure on the lower arm.

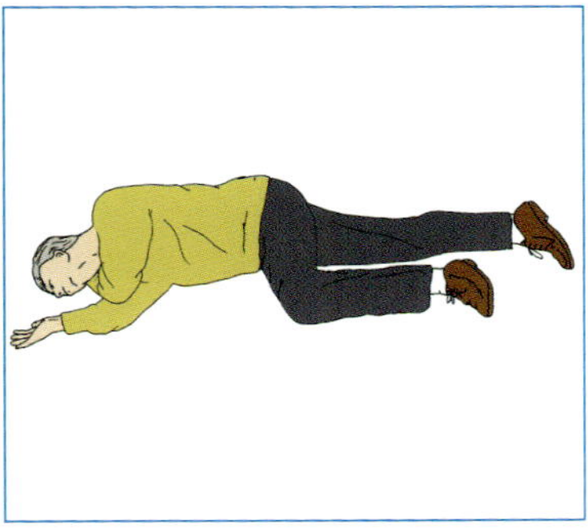

Figure 2.17. The recovery position. © ERC 2005.

Foreign body airway obstruction (choking)

Foreign body airway obstruction (FBAO) is an uncommon but potentially treatable cause of accidental death. As most choking events are associated with eating, it is a commonly witnessed event. As such, there is often the opportunity for early intervention while the victim is still responsive.

Recognition

Because recognition of airway obstruction is the key to successful outcome, it is important not to confuse this emergency with fainting, heart attack, seizure or other conditions that may cause sudden respiratory distress, cyanosis or loss of consciousness.

Foreign bodies may cause either mild or severe airway obstruction. The signs and symptoms enabling differentiation between mild and severe airway obstruction are summarised in Table 2.1. It is important to ask the conscious victim "Are you choking?"

Table 2.1 Differentiation between mild and severe FBAO

General signs of FBAO	
• Attack occurs while eating • Victim may clutch his neck	
Signs of mild airway obstruction	**Signs of severe airway obstruction**
Response to question "Are you choking?": • Victim speaks and answers yes	Response to question "Are you choking?": • Victim unable to speak • Victim may respond by nodding
Other signs: • Victim is able to speak, cough and breathe	Other signs: • Victim unable to breathe • Breathing sounds wheezy • Attempts at coughing are silent • Victim may be unconscious

Adult FBAO (choking) sequence (Figure 2.18)

This sequence is also suitable for use in children over the age of 1 y).

1. **If the victim shows signs of mild airway obstruction:**
   - Encourage him to continue coughing but do nothing else.
2. **If the victim shows signs of severe airway obstruction:**
   If the victim is conscious:
   - Apply up to five back blows:
     - Stand to the side and slightly behind the victim.
     - Support the chest with one hand and lean the victim well forwards so that when the obstructing object is dislodged it comes out of the mouth rather than goes further down the airway.
     - Give up to five sharp blows between the shoulder blades with the heel of your other hand.
   - Check to see if each back blow has relieved the airway obstruction. The aim is to relieve the obstruction with each blow rather than necessarily to give all five.
   - If five back blows fail to relieve the airway obstruction give up to five abdominal thrusts:

  - Stand behind the victim and put both arms round the upper part of his abdomen.
  - Lean the victim forwards.
  - Clench your fist and place it between the umbilicus and xiphisternum.
  - Grasp this hand with your other hand and pull sharply inwards and upwards.
  - Repeat up to five times.
- If the obstruction is still not relieved continue alternating five back blows with five abdominal thrusts.

If the victim at any time becomes unconscious:

- Support the victim carefully to the ground.
- Immediately activate EMS.
- Begin CPR (from 5B of the adult BLS sequence). Healthcare providers, trained and experienced in feeling for a carotid pulse, should initiate chest compressions, even if a pulse is present in the unconscious choking victim.

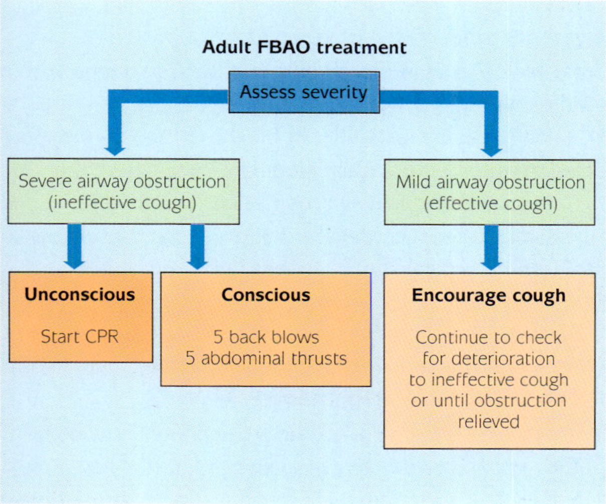

Figure 2.18. Algorithm for choking in adults.

FBAO with severe airway obstruction

For conscious adults and children over 1 y with a complete FBAO, the likelihood of successful relief is increased when combinations of back blows or slaps, and abdominal and chest thrusts, are used.

Unconscious victim

Higher airway pressures can be generated using chest thrusts compared with abdominal thrusts. Since chest thrusts are virtually identical to chest compressions, rescuers should start CPR if a victim of known or suspected FBAO becomes unconscious. During CPR, each time the airway is opened the victim's mouth should be quickly checked for any foreign body that has been partly expelled.

The incidence of unsuspected choking as a cause of unconsciousness or cardiac arrest is low; therefore, during CPR routinely checking the mouth for foreign bodies is not necessary. Blind finger sweeps can cause harm to the victim or rescuer and should be avoided. Only if solid material can be seen in the airway should it be removed manually.

Aftercare and referral for medical review

Following successful treatment for FBAO, victims with a persistent cough, difficulty swallowing, or with the sensation of an object being still stuck in the throat, should therefore be referred for a medical opinion.

Abdominal thrusts can cause serious internal injuries and all victims treated with abdominal thrusts should be examined for injury by a doctor.

Resuscitation of children (see also Chapter 5) and victims of drowning (see also Chapter 6)

Both ventilation and compression are important for victims of cardiac arrest when the oxygen stores become depleted – about 4–6 min after collapse from VF and immediately after collapse for victims of asphyxial arrest. Previous guidelines tried to take into account the difference in pathophysiology and recommended that victims of identifiable asphyxia (drowning, trauma, intoxication) and children should receive 1 min of CPR before the lone rescuer left the victim to get help. The majority of cases of SCA out of hospital, however, occur in adults and are of cardiac origin due to VF. These additional recommendations, therefore, added to the complexity of the guidelines whilst affecting only a minority of victims.

Also important is that many children do not receive resuscitation because potential rescuers fear causing harm. This fear is unfounded; it is far better to use the adult BLS sequence for resuscitation of a child than to do nothing.

For ease of teaching and retention, therefore, lay people should be taught that the adult sequence may also be used for children who are not responsive and not breathing.

The following minor modifications to the adult sequence will, however, make it even more suitable for use in children:

- Give five initial rescue breaths before starting chest compressions (adult sequence of actions, see pages 17–19).
- A lone rescuer should perform CPR for approximately 1 min before going for help.
- Compress the chest by approximately one-third of its depth; use two fingers for an infant under 1 y; use one or two hands for children less than 8 y, according to rescuer preference, to achieve an adequate depth of compression.

The same modifications of five initial breaths, and 1 min of CPR by the lone rescuer before getting help, may improve outcome for victims of drowning. This modification should be taught only to those who have a specific duty of care to potential drowning victims (e.g. lifeguards).

Drowning is easily identified. It can be difficult, on the other hand, for a lay person to determine whether cardiorespiratory arrest is a direct result of trauma or intoxication. These victims should, therefore, be managed according to the standard protocol.

Use of an automated external defibrillator (AED)

Chapter 3 discusses the guidelines for defibrillation using both automated external defibrillators (AEDs) and manual defibrillators, but there are some special considerations when an AED is to be used by lay or non-healthcare rescuers.

Standard AEDs are suitable for use in children older than 8 y. In children between 1 and 8 y, use paediatric pads or a paediatric mode if available; if not, use the AED as it is. Use of AEDs is not recommended in children less than 1 y.

Sequence for use of an AED (Figure 2.19)

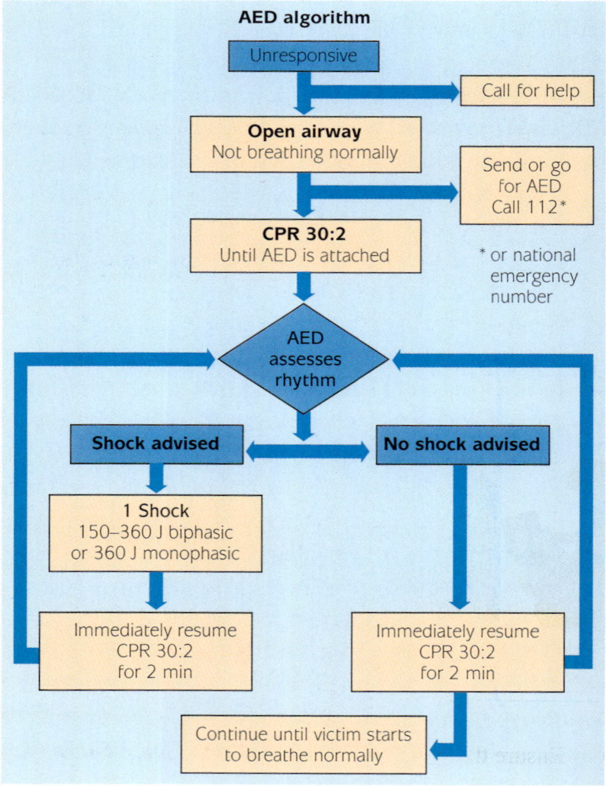

Figure 2.19. Algorithm for AED.

1. **Make sure you, the victim and any bystanders are safe.**
2. **If the victim is unresponsive and not breathing normally:**
- Send someone for the AED and call for an ambulance.
3. **Start CPR according to the guidelines for BLS.**
4. **As soon as the defibrillator arrives:**
- Switch on the defibrillator (Figure 2.20) and attach the electrode pads.

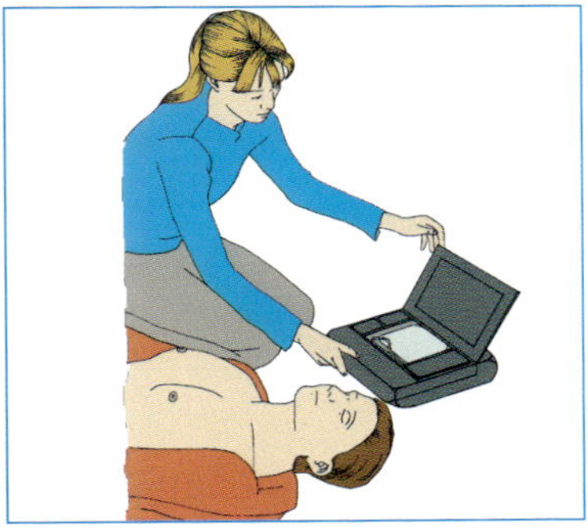

Figure 2.20. Switch on the defibrillator. © ERC 2005.

- If more than one rescuer is present, CPR should be continued whilst this is done (Figure 2.21).
- Follow the spoken/visual directions.

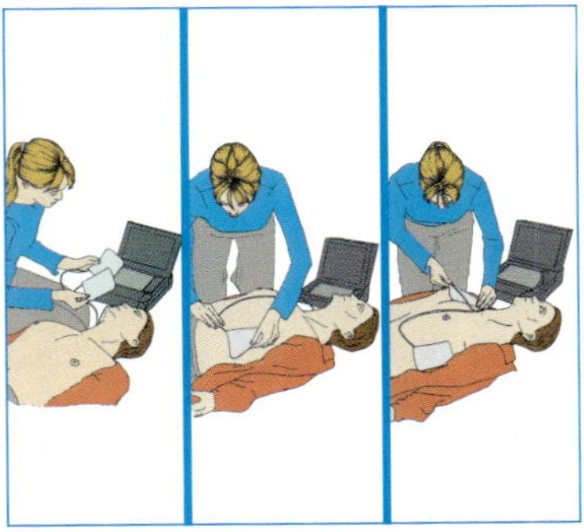

Figure 2.21. Attach the electrode pads. © ERC 2005.

- Ensure that nobody touches the victim whilst the AED is analysing the rhythm (Figure 2.22).

5A. If a shock *IS* indicated:

- Ensure that nobody touches the victim.
- Push shock button as directed (fully automatic AEDs will deliver the shock automatically).
- Continue as directed by the voice/visual prompts.

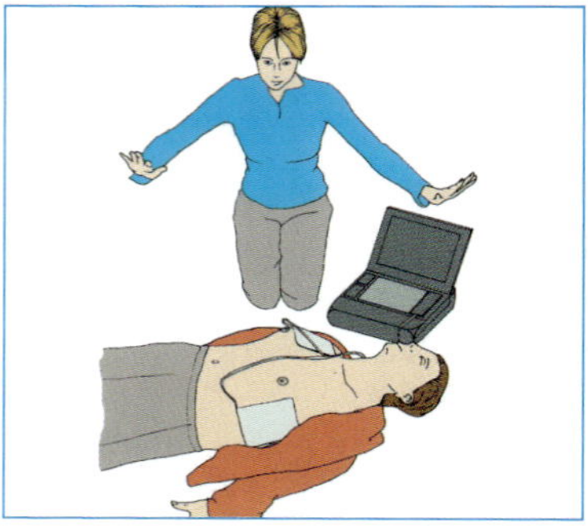

Figure 2.22. Ensure that nobody touches the victim. © ERC 2005.

5B. If *NO* shock is indicated:

- Immediately resume CPR using a ratio of 30 compressions to two rescue breaths.
- Continue as directed by the voice/visual prompts.

6. Continue to follow the AED prompts until:

- Qualified help arrives and takes over.
- The victim starts to breathe normally.
- You become exhausted.

CPR before defibrillation

Immediate defibrillation, as soon as an AED becomes available, has always been a key element in guidelines and teaching, and considered of paramount importance for survival from ventricular fibrillation. This concept has been challenged because evidence suggests that a period of chest compression before defibrillation may improve survival when the time between calling for the ambulance and its arrival exceeds 5 min. However, in all the studies, CPR was performed by paramedics who protected the airway by intubation and delivered 100% oxygen. It is also unlikely, in the majority of cases of out-of-hospital cardiac arrest, that the delay from collapse to arrival of the rescuer with an AED will be known with certainty. For these reasons, these guidelines recommend an immediate shock, as soon as the AED is available. The importance of early uninterrupted external chest compression is emphasised.

The shock sequence and energy levels are discussed in Chapter 3.

Fully-automatic AEDs

Having detected a shockable rhythm, a fully-automatic AED will deliver a shock without further input from the rescuer. One manikin study showed that untrained nursing students committed fewer safety errors using a fully-automatic AED rather than a semi-automatic AED. There are no human data to determine whether these findings can be applied to clinical use.

Further reading

1. International Liaison Committee on Resuscitation. 2005 International Consensus on Cardiopulmonary Resuscitation and Emergency Cardiovascular Care Science with Treatment Recommendations. Resuscitation 2005;67:187–211.
2. European Resuscitation Council. European Resuscitation Council guidelines for resuscitation 2005. Resuscitation 2005;67(Suppl 1):S7–23, S25–37.

Chapter 3
Advanced life support

Charles D Deakin, Jerry P Nolan, Jasmeet Soar, Bernd W Böttiger and Gary Smith

Introduction

The 2005 ERC ALS guidelines adhere to the same general principles as previous guidelines, but incorporate some important changes, particularly in relation to defibrillation, the timing of defibrillation in relation to external chest compression, the number of shocks that should be delivered and the recommendations for defibrillation energy. With outcome from cardiac arrest so poor, there is also greater emphasis on the recognition and prevention of cardiac arrest. For patients in whom a spontaneous circulation is restored more in-depth guidelines are given for post-resuscitation care.

Prevention of in-hospital cardiac arrest

Approximately 80% of cardiac arrests in hospital are preceded by a slow and progressive physiological deterioration. Early and effective treatment of seriously ill patients might prevent some cardiac arrests, deaths and unanticipated ICU admissions. The deficiencies in acute care are related to lack of acute care knowledge and skills across all grades of clinical staff. To improve the identification of patients at risk of cardiac arrest, many hospitals now use early warning scores (EWS) that identify risk according to the extent of derangement of several physiological parameters. Alternatively, response for assistance may be triggered when one or more variables of routine observations cross a predetermined threshold. The benefits of one system over the other have not been established, although the EWS methodology has the advantage of tracking changes in physiology and warning of impending physiological collapse instead of waiting until an extreme value of physiology has been reached. Both methods rely on accurate recording of patient vital signs and prompt action when abnormalities are detected.

Many hospitals have introduced a medical emergency team (MET) or outreach team that responds to patients with acute physiological deterioration as well as those in cardiac arrest. The benefit of these teams in reducing the incidence of cardiac arrest, unexpected death or unplanned ICU admission remains to be proven.

The following strategies may prevent avoidable in-hospital cardiac arrests:

1. Treat patients who are critically ill or at risk of clinical deterioration in appropriate areas, matching the level of care to sickness severity.
2. Critically ill patients need regular observations to match the frequency and type of observations to the severity of illness or the likelihood of clinical deterioration and cardiopulmonary arrest. Often only simple vital sign observations (pulse, blood pressure, respiratory rate) are needed.
3. Use an EWS system linked to an appropriate clinical response to identify patients who are critically ill or at risk of clinical deterioration and cardiopulmonary arrest.
4. Train all clinical staff in the recognition, monitoring and initial treatment of the critically ill patient.
5. Identify:

- Patients for whom cardiopulmonary arrest is an anticipated terminal event and in whom CPR is inappropriate.
- Patients who do not wish to be treated with CPR. Hospitals should have a do not attempt resuscitation (DNAR) policy based on existing national guidance.

In-hospital resuscitation

For all in-hospital cardiac arrests, ensure that:

- Cardiorespiratory arrest is recognised immediately.
- Help is summoned using a standard telephone number.

- CPR is started immediately using effective chest compressions, airway adjuncts, e.g. a pocket mask, and, if indicated, defibrillation attempted within 3 min.

All healthcare professionals should be able to recognise cardiac arrest, call for help and start CPR. The single responder must ensure that help is coming. All clinical areas should have immediate access to resuscitation equipment and drugs to facilitate rapid resuscitation of the patient in cardiopulmonary arrest. Ideally, the equipment used for cardiopulmonary resuscitation (including defibrillators) and the layout of equipment and drugs should be standardised throughout the hospital.

Immediate actions for 'collapsed' patient in a hospital

An algorithm for the initial management of in-hospital cardiac arrest is shown in Figure 3.1.

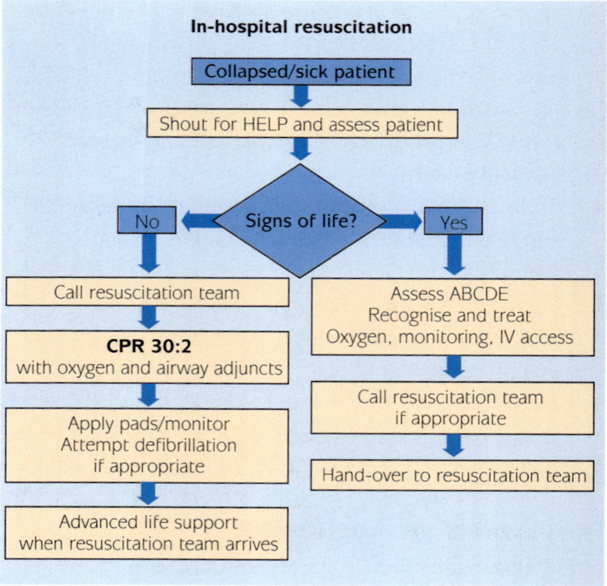

Figure 3.1. Algorithm for the treatment of in-hospital cardiac arrest.

1. **Ensure personal safety.**
2. **Check the victim for a response:**

- When a healthcare professional sees a patient collapse or finds a patient apparently unconscious in a clinical area they should first shout for help, then assess if the patient is responsive (shake and shout).*
- If other members of staff are nearby it will be possible to undertake actions simultaneously.

  * Gently shake his shoulders and ask loudly: "Are you all right?"

The responsive patient

Urgent medical assessment is required. Depending on the local protocols, this may take the form of a resuscitation team (e.g. MET). While awaiting this team, give the patient oxygen, attach monitoring and insert an intravenous cannula.

The unresponsive patient

The exact sequence will depend on the training of staff and experience in assessment of breathing and circulation. Trained healthcare staff cannot assess the breathing and pulse sufficiently reliably to confirm cardiac arrest. Agonal breathing (occasional gasps, slow, laboured or noisy breathing) is common in the early stages of cardiac arrest and is a sign of cardiac arrest and should not be confused as a sign of life/circulation.

1. **Shout for help** (if not already).
   Turn the victim on to his back and then open the airway:
2. **Open airway and check breathing.**

- Open the airway using a head tilt/chin lift.
- Look in the mouth. If a foreign body or debris is visible attempt to remove with a finger sweep, forceps or suction as appropriate.
- If you suspect that there may have been an injury to the neck, try to open the airway using jaw thrust or chin lift without head tilt. Remember that maintaining an airway and adequate ventilation is the overriding priority in managing a patient with a suspected spinal injury. If this is unsuccessful, use just enough head tilt to clear the

airway. Use manual in-line stabilisation to minimise head movement if sufficient rescuers are available.

Keeping the airway open, look, listen and feel for normal breathing (an occasional gasp, slow, laboured or noisy breathing is not normal):

- Look for chest movement.
- Listen at the victim's mouth for breath sounds.
- Feel for air on your cheek.

Look, listen and feel for no more than **10 s** to determine if the victim is breathing normally.

3. **Check for signs of a circulation.**

- It may be difficult to be certain that there is no pulse. If the patient has no signs of life (lack of movement, normal breathing or coughing), start CPR until more experienced help arrives or the patient shows signs of life.
- Those experienced in clinical assessment should assess the carotid pulse whilst simultaneously looking for signs of life for not more than 10 s.
- If the patient appears to have no signs of life, or if there is doubt, start CPR immediately. Delays in diagnosis of cardiac arrest and starting CPR, which will adversely affect survival, must be avoided.

If there is a pulse or signs of life urgent medical assessment is required. Depending on the local protocols, this may take the form of a resuscitation team. While awaiting the arrival of this team, give the patient oxygen, attach monitoring and insert an intravenous cannula.

If there is no breathing, but there is a pulse (respiratory arrest), ventilate the patient's lungs and check for a circulation every 10–12 breaths.

Starting in-hospital cardiopulmonary resuscitation

- One person starts CPR as others call the resuscitation team and collect the resuscitation equipment and a defibrillator. If only one member of staff is present, this will mean leaving the patient.

- Give 30 chest compressions followed by two ventilations.
- Undertaking chest compressions properly is tiring; try to change the person doing chest compressions every 2 min.
- Maintain the airway and ventilate the lungs with the most appropriate equipment immediately at hand. A pocket mask, which may be supplemented with an oral airway, is usually readily available. Alternatively, use a laryngeal mask airway (LMA) and self-inflating bag, or bag-mask, according to local policy. Tracheal intubation should be attempted only by those who are trained, competent and experienced in this skill.
- Use an inspiratory time of 1 s and give enough volume to produce a normal chest rise. Add supplemental oxygen as soon as possible.
- Once the patient's trachea has been intubated, continue chest compressions uninterrupted (except for defibrillation or pulse checks when indicated), at a rate of 100 min^{-1}, and ventilate the lungs at approximately 10 breaths min^{-1}. Avoid hyperventilation.
- If there is no airway and ventilation equipment available, give mouth-to-mouth ventilation. If there are clinical reasons to avoid mouth-to-mouth contact, or you are unwilling or unable to do this, do chest compressions until help or airway equipment arrives.
- When the defibrillator arrives, apply the paddles to the patient and analyse the rhythm. If self-adhesive defibrillation pads are available, apply these without interrupting chest compressions. Pause briefly to assess the heart rhythm. If indicated, attempt either manual or automated external defibrillation (AED).
- Recommence chest compressions immediately after the defibrillation attempt. Minimise interruptions to chest compressions.
- Continue resuscitation until the resuscitation team arrives or the patient shows signs of life. Follow the voice prompts if using an AED. If using a manual

defibrillator follow the universal algorithm for advanced life support.

- Once resuscitation is underway, and if there are sufficient people, prepare intravenous cannulae and drugs likely to be used by the resuscitation team (e.g. adrenaline).
- Identify one person to be responsible for hand-over to the resuscitation team leader. Locate the patient's records.
- The quality of chest compressions during in-hospital CPR is frequently sub-optimal. The team leader should monitor the quality of CPR and use an alternate CPR provider if the quality of chest compressions is poor. The person providing chest compressions should be alternated every 2 min.

The monitored and witnessed cardiac arrest

If a patient has a monitored and witnessed cardiac arrest:

- Confirm cardiac arrest and shout for help.
- Consider a precordial thump if the rhythm is ventricular fibrillation/pulseless VT (VF/VT) and a defibrillator is not immediately available.
- If the initial rhythm is VF/VT and a defibrillator is immediately available, give a shock first. The use of adhesive electrode pads or the 'quick look' paddles technique will enable rapid assessment of heart rhythm compared with attaching ECG electrodes.

ALS treatment algorithm

Heart rhythms associated with cardiac arrest are divided into two groups: shockable rhythms (VF/VT) and non-shockable rhythms [asystole and pulseless electrical activity (PEA)]. The principle difference in the treatment of these two groups of arrhythmias is the need for attempted defibrillation in those patients with VF/VT. Subsequent actions, including chest compressions, airway management and ventilation, venous access, administration of adrenaline and the identification and correction of reversible factors, are common to both groups.

Although the ALS cardiac arrest algorithm (Figure 3.2) is applicable to all cardiac arrests, additional interventions may be indicated for cardiac arrest caused by special circumstances.

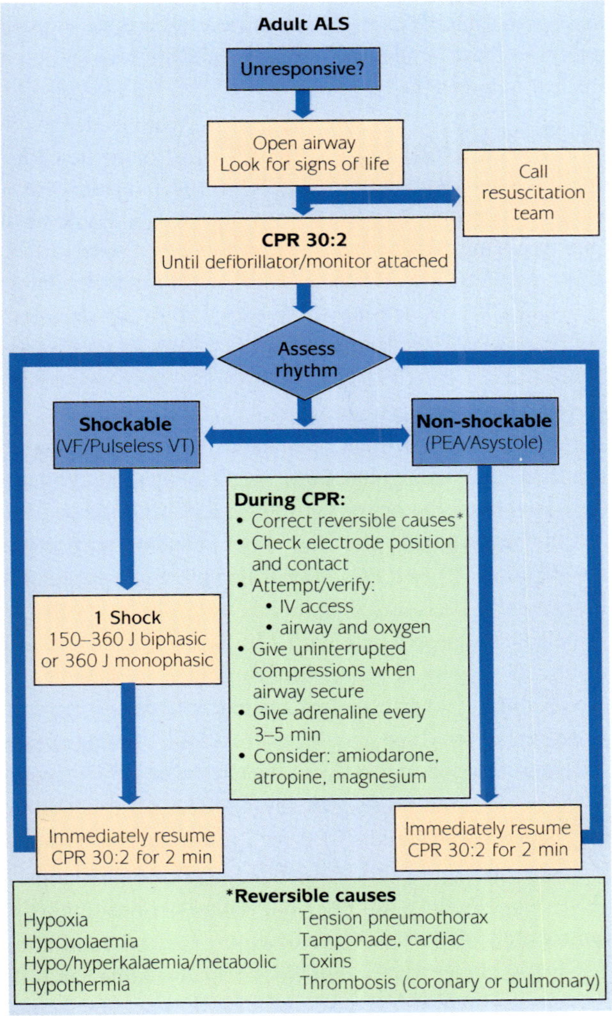

Figure 3.2. Advanced life support cardiac arrest algorithm.

The interventions that contribute unquestionably to improved survival after cardiac arrest are early defibrillation for VF/VT and prompt and effective bystander basic life support (BLS). Advanced airway intervention and the delivery of drugs have not been shown to increase survival to hospital discharge after cardiac arrest, although they are still included among ALS interventions. Thus, during advanced life support, attention must be focused on early defibrillation and high quality, uninterrupted BLS.

Shockable rhythms (VF/VT)

In adults, the commonest rhythm at the time of cardiac arrest is VF, which may be preceded by a period of VT or even supraventricular tachycardia (SVT). Having confirmed cardiac arrest, summon help (including a request for a defibrillator) and start CPR, beginning with external chest compression, with a compression:ventilation ratio of 30:2. As soon as the defibrillator arrives, diagnose the rhythm by applying paddles or self-adhesive pads to the chest.

If VF/VT is confirmed, charge the defibrillator and give one shock (150–200 J biphasic or 360 J monophasic). Without reassessing the rhythm or feeling for a pulse, resume CPR (30:2), immediately after the shock, starting with chest compressions. Even if the defibrillation attempt is successful in restoring a perfusing rhythm, it is very rare for a pulse to be palpable immediately after defibrillation and the delay in trying to palpate a pulse will further compromise the myocardium if a perfusing rhythm has not been restored. If a perfusing rhythm has been restored, giving chest compressions does not increase the chance of VF recurring. In the presence of post-shock asystole chest compressions may induce VF. Continue CPR for 2 min, then pause briefly to check the monitor: if still VF/VT, give a second shock (150–360 J biphasic or 360 J monophasic). Resume CPR immediately after the second shock.

Pause briefly after 2 min of CPR to check the monitor: if there is still VF/VT, give adrenaline followed immediately by a third shock (150–360 J biphasic or 360 J monophasic) and resumption of CPR (**drug–shock–CPR–rhythm check sequence**). Minimise the delay between stopping chest compressions and delivery of the shock. The adrenaline that is given immediately before the shock will be circulated by the CPR that immediately follows the shock. After drug delivery and 2 min of CPR, analyse the rhythm and be prepared to deliver another shock immediately if indicated. If VF/VT persists after the third shock, give an intravenous bolus of amiodarone 300 mg. Inject the amiodarone during the brief rhythm analysis before delivery of the fourth shock.

When the rhythm is checked 2 min after giving a shock, if a non-shockable rhythm is present and the rhythm is organised (complexes appear regular or narrow), try to palpate a pulse. Rhythm checks must be brief, and pulse checks undertaken only if an organised rhythm is observed. If an organised rhythm is seen during a 2 min period of CPR, do not interrupt chest compressions to palpate a pulse unless the patient shows signs of life suggesting ROSC. If there is any doubt about the presence of a pulse in the presence of an organised rhythm, resume CPR. If the patient has ROSC, begin post-resuscitation care. If the patient's rhythm changes to asystole or PEA, see non-shockable rhythms below.

During treatment of VF/VT, healthcare providers must practise efficient coordination between CPR and shock delivery. When VF is present for more than a few minutes, the myocardium is depleted of oxygen and metabolic substrates. A brief period of chest compressions will deliver oxygen and energy substrates and increase the probability of restoring a perfusing rhythm after shock delivery. Analyses of VF waveform characteristics predictive of shock success indicate that the shorter the time between chest compression and shock delivery, the more likely the shock will be successful. Reduction in the interval from compression to shock delivery by even a few seconds can increase the probability of shock success.

Regardless of the arrest rhythm, give adrenaline 1 mg every 3–5 min until ROSC is achieved; this will be once every two loops of the algorithm. If signs of life return during CPR (movement, normal breathing or coughing), check the monitor: if an organised rhythm is present, check for a pulse. If a pulse is palpable, continue post-resuscitation care and/or treatment of peri-arrest arrhythmia. If no pulse is present, continue CPR. Providing CPR with a CV ratio of 30:2 is tiring; change the individual undertaking compressions every 2 min.

Precordial thump

Consider giving a single precordial thump when cardiac arrest is confirmed rapidly after a witnessed, sudden collapse and a defibrillator is not immediately to hand. These circumstances are most likely to occur when the patient is monitored. A precordial thump should be undertaken immediately after confirmation of cardiac arrest and only by healthcare professionals trained in the technique. Using the ulnar edge of a tightly clenched fist, deliver a sharp impact to the lower half of the sternum from a height of about 20 cm, then retract the fist immediately to create an impulse-like stimulus. A precordial thump is most likely to be successful in converting VT to sinus rhythm. Successful treatment of VF by precordial thump is much less likely: in all the reported successful cases the precordial thump was given within the first 10 s of VF. There are very rare reports of a precordial thump converting a perfusing to a non-perfusing rhythm.

Airway and ventilation

During the treatment of persistent VF, ensure good quality chest compressions between defibrillation attempts. Consider reversible causes (four Hs and four Ts) and, if identified, correct them. Check the electrode/defibrillating paddle positions and contacts, and the adequacy of the coupling medium, e.g. gel pads. Tracheal intubation provides the most reliable airway but should be attempted only if the healthcare provider is properly trained and has adequate ongoing experience with the technique. Personnel skilled in advanced airway management should attempt laryngoscopy without stopping chest compressions – a brief pause in chest compressions may be required as the tube is passed through the vocal cords. Alternatively, to avoid any interruptions in chest compressions, the intubation attempt may be deferred until return of spontaneous circulation. No intubation attempt should take longer than 30 s: if intubation has not been achieved after this time, recommence bag-mask ventilation. After intubation, confirm correct tube position and secure it adequately. Once the patient's trachea has been intubated, continue chest compressions, at a rate of 100 min^{-1}, without pausing during ventilation. Ventilate the lungs at 10 breaths min^{-1}. Do not hyperventilate the patient. A pause in the chest compressions allows the coronary perfusion pressure to fall substantially. On resuming compressions there is some delay before the original coronary perfusion pressure is restored; thus, chest compressions uninterrupted for ventilation result in a substantially higher mean coronary perfusion pressure.

In the absence of personnel skilled in tracheal intubation, acceptable alternatives are the Combitube, laryngeal mask airway (LMA), ProSeal LMA or laryngeal tube. Once one of these airways has been inserted, attempt to deliver continuous chest compressions, uninterrupted during ventilation. If excessive gas leakage causes inadequate ventilation of the patient's lungs, chest compressions will have to be interrupted to enable ventilation (using a ratio of 30 compressions to two ventilations).

During continuous chest compressions, ventilate the lungs at 10 breaths min^{-1}.

Intravenous access and drugs

Peripheral versus central venous drug delivery

Establish intravenous access if this has not already been achieved. Although peak drug concentrations are higher and circulation times are shorter when drugs are injected into a central venous catheter compared with a peripheral cannula, insertion of a central venous catheter requires interruption of CPR and is associated with several complications. Peripheral venous cannulation is quicker, easier to perform and safer.

Drugs injected peripherally must be followed by a flush of at least 20 ml of fluid and elevation of the extremity for 10–20 s to facilitate drug delivery to the central circulation.

Intraosseous route

If intravenous access is difficult or impossible, consider the intraosseous route. Although normally considered as an alternative route for vascular access in children, it can also be effective in adults. Intraosseous injection of drugs achieves adequate plasma concentrations in a time comparable to injection through a central venous catheter. The intraosseous route also enables withdrawal of marrow for venous blood gas analysis and measurement of electrolytes and haemoglobin concentration.

Tracheal route

If intravenous and intraosseous access cannot be established, some drugs can be given by the tracheal route. However, unpredictable plasma concentrations are achieved when drugs are given via a tracheal tube and the optimal tracheal dose of most drugs is unknown. During CPR, the equipotent dose of adrenaline given via the trachea is 3–10 times higher than the intravenous dose. Some animal studies suggest that the lower adrenaline concentrations achieved when the drug is given via the trachea may produce transient α-adrenergic effects, which will cause hypotension and a decrease in coronary artery perfusion pressure.

If given via the trachea, the dose of adrenaline is 3 mg diluted to at least 10 ml with sterile water. Dilution with water instead of 0.9% saline may achieve better drug absorption. The solutions in prefilled syringes are acceptable for this purpose.

Adrenaline

Despite the widespread use of adrenaline during resuscitation and several studies involving vasopressin, there is no placebo-controlled study that shows that the routine use of any vasopressor at any stage during human cardiac arrest increases survival to hospital discharge. Current evidence is insufficient to support or refute the routine use of any particular drug or sequence of drugs. Despite the lack of human data the use of adrenaline is still recommended, based largely on animal data. The α-adrenergic actions of adrenaline cause vasoconstriction, which increases myocardial and cerebral perfusion pressure. The higher coronary blood flow increases the frequency of the VF waveform and should improve the chance of restoring a circulation when defibrillation is attempted. The optimal duration of CPR and number of shocks that should be delivered before giving drugs are unknown. On the basis of expert consensus, if VF/VT persists after two shocks, give adrenaline and repeat every 3–5 min during cardiac arrest. Do not interrupt CPR to give drugs.

Vasopressin

A recent meta-analysis of five randomised trials showed no statistically significant difference between vasopressin and adrenaline for ROSC, death within 24 h or death before hospital discharge. The sub-group analysis based on initial cardiac rhythm did not show any statistically significant difference in the rate of death before hospital discharge. Despite the absence of placebo-controlled trials, adrenaline has been the standard vasopressor in cardiac arrest. There is insufficient evidence to support or refute the use of vasopressin as an alternative to, or in combination with, adrenaline in any cardiac arrest rhythm. Thus, adrenaline remains as the primary vasopressor for the treatment of cardiac arrest of all rhythms.

Anti-arrhythmic drugs

There is no evidence that giving any anti-arrhythmic drug routinely during human cardiac arrest increases survival to hospital discharge. In comparison with placebo and lidocaine, the use of amiodarone in shock refractory VF improves the short-term outcome of survival to hospital admission. In these studies, the anti-arrhythmic therapy was given if VF/VT persisted after at least three shocks; however, these were delivered using the conventional three-stacked shocks strategy. There are no data on the use of amiodarone for shock refractory VF/VT when single shocks are used. On the basis of expert consensus, if VF/VT persists after three shocks, give amiodarone 300 mg by bolus injection. A further dose of 150 mg may be given for recurrent or refractory VF/VT, followed by an infusion of 900 mg over 24 h. Lidocaine 1 mg kg^{-1} may be used as an alternative if amiodarone is not available, but do not give lidocaine if amiodarone has been given already.

Magnesium

Although the routine use of magnesium in cardiac arrest does not increase survival, give magnesium [8 mmol = 4 ml 50% magnesium sulphate (2 g)] for refractory VF if there is any suspicion of hypomagnesaemia (e.g. patients on potassium-losing diuretics).

Bicarbonate

Giving sodium bicarbonate routinely during cardiac arrest and CPR (especially in out-of-hospital cardiac arrests) or after return of spontaneous circulation is not recommended. Give sodium bicarbonate (50 mmol) if cardiac arrest is associated with hyperkalaemia or tricyclic antidepressant overdose; repeat the dose according to the clinical condition and result of repeated blood gas analysis. Some experts give bicarbonate if the arterial pH is less than 7.1, but this is controversial. During cardiac arrest, arterial blood gas values do not reflect the acid–base state of the tissues. During cardiac arrest the tissue pH will be lower than that in arterial blood. Mixed venous blood values give a more accurate estimate of the pH in the tissues but it is rare for a pulmonary artery catheter to be in situ at the time of cardiac arrest. If a central venous catheter is in situ, central venous blood gas analysis will provide a closer estimate of tissue acid–base state than that provided by arterial blood.

Persistent ventricular fibrillation

If VF persists, consider changing the position of the paddles (see page 56). Review all potentially reversible causes (see below) and treat any that are identified.

The duration of any individual resuscitation attempt is a matter of clinical judgement, taking into consideration the circumstances and the perceived prospect of a successful outcome. If it was considered appropriate to start resuscitation, it is usually considered worthwhile continuing as long as the patient remains in VF/VT.

Non-shockable rhythms (PEA and asystole)

Pulseless electrical activity (PEA) is defined as cardiac electrical activity in the absence of any palpable pulses. These patients often have some mechanical myocardial contractions but they are too weak to produce a detectable pulse or blood pressure. PEA is often caused by reversible conditions and can be treated if those conditions are identified and corrected (see below). Survival following cardiac arrest with asystole or PEA is unlikely unless a reversible cause can be found and treated effectively.

If the initial monitored rhythm is PEA or asystole, start CPR 30:2 and give adrenaline 1 mg as soon as intravascular access is achieved. If asystole is displayed, without stopping CPR, check that the leads are attached correctly. Asystole is a condition that could be exacerbated or precipitated by excessive vagal tone and, theoretically, this could be reversed by a vagolytic drug; therefore, despite the lack of evidence that giving routinely for asystolic cardiac arrest increases survival, give atropine 3 mg (the dose that will provide maximum vagal blockade) if there is asystole or the rhythm is slow PEA (rate <60 min^{-1}). Secure the airway as soon as possible to enable chest compressions to be delivered without pausing during ventilation. After 2 min of CPR, recheck the rhythm. If no rhythm is present (asystole) or if there is no change in the ECG appearance, resume CPR immediately. If an organised rhythm is present, attempt to palpate a pulse. If no pulse is present (or if there is any doubt about the presence of a pulse), continue CPR. If a pulse is present, begin post-resuscitation care. If signs of life return during CPR, check the rhythm and attempt to palpate a pulse.

Whenever a diagnosis of asystole is made, check the ECG carefully for the presence of P waves because this may respond to cardiac pacing. There is no benefit in attempting to pace true asystole.

If there is doubt about whether the rhythm is asystole or fine VF, do not attempt defibrillation; instead, continue chest compressions and ventilation. Fine VF that is difficult to distinguish from asystole will not be shocked successfully into a perfusing rhythm. Continuing good quality CPR may improve the amplitude and frequency of the VF and improve the chance of successful defibrillation to a perfusing rhythm. Delivering repeated shocks in an attempt to defibrillate what is thought to be fine VF will increase myocardial injury both directly from the electricity and indirectly from the interruptions in coronary blood flow.

During the treatment of asystole or PEA, if the rhythm changes to VF, follow the left side of the algorithm. Otherwise, continue CPR and give adrenaline every 3–5 min (every other loop of the algorithm).

Potentially reversible causes

Potential causes or aggravating factors for which specific treatment exists must be considered during any cardiac arrest. For ease of memory, these are divided into two groups of four, based upon their initial letter – either H or T. More details on many of these conditions are covered in Chapter 6.

The four 'Hs'

Minimise the risk of **hypoxia** by ensuring that the patient's lungs are ventilated adequately with 100% oxygen. Make sure there is adequate chest rise and bilateral breath sounds. Using the techniques described below, check carefully that the tracheal tube is not misplaced in a bronchus or the oesophagus.

Pulseless electrical activity caused by **hypovolaemia** is usually due to severe haemorrhage. This may be precipitated by trauma, gastrointestinal bleeding or rupture of an aortic aneurysm. Intravascular volume should be restored rapidly with fluid, coupled with urgent surgery to stop the haemorrhage.

Hyperkalaemia, hypokalaemia, hypocalcaemia, acidaemia and other metabolic disorders are detected by biochemical tests or suggested by the patient's medical history, e.g. renal failure. A 12-lead ECG may be diagnostic. Intravenous calcium chloride is indicated in the presence of hyperkalaemia, hypocalcaemia and calcium channel-blocker overdose.

Suspect **hypothermia** in any drowning or exposure incident; use a low reading thermometer.

The four 'Ts'

A **tension pneumothorax** may be the primary cause of PEA and may follow attempts at central venous catheter insertion. The diagnosis is made clinically. Decompress rapidly by needle thoracocentesis, and then insert a chest drain.

Cardiac **tamponade** is difficult to diagnose because the typical signs of distended neck veins and hypotension are usually obscured by the arrest itself. Cardiac arrest after penetrating chest trauma is highly suggestive of tamponade and is an indication for needle pericardiocentesis or resuscitative thoracotomy.

In the absence of a specific history, the accidental or deliberate ingestion of therapeutic or **toxic** substances may be revealed only by laboratory investigations. Where available, the appropriate antidotes should be used but most often treatment is supportive.

The commonest cause of **thromboembolic** or mechanical circulatory obstruction is massive pulmonary embolus. If cardiac arrest is thought to be caused by pulmonary embolism consider giving a thrombolytic drug immediately. Thrombolysis may be considered in adult cardiac arrest on a case-by-case basis following initial failure of standard resuscitation in patients in whom an acute thrombotic aetiology for the arrest is suspected. Ongoing CPR is not a contraindication to thrombolysis.

Calcium

Calcium is indicated during resuscitation from PEA thought to be caused by:

- Hyperkalaemia.
- Hypocalcaemia.
- Overdose of calcium channel-blocking drugs.

The initial dose of 10 ml 10% calcium chloride (6.8 mmol Ca^{2+}) may be repeated if necessary. Calcium can slow the heart rate and precipitate arrhythmias. In cardiac arrest, calcium may be given by rapid intravenous injection. In the presence of a spontaneous circulation give it slowly. Do not give calcium solutions and sodium bicarbonate simultaneously by the same route.

Intravenous fluids

Hypovolaemia is a potentially reversible cause of cardiac arrest – infuse fluids rapidly if hypovolaemia is suspected. In the initial stages of resuscitation there are no clear advantages to using colloid. Use saline or Hartmann's solution. Avoid dextrose – this is redistributed away from the intravascular space rapidly and causes hyperglycaemia, which may worsen neurological outcome after cardiac arrest.

Open chest CPR

Open chest CPR may be indicated for patients with cardiac arrest due to trauma, in the early post-operative phase after cardiothoracic surgery or when the chest or abdomen is already open – for example, in trauma surgery.

Defibrillation

The benefits of early defibrillation have led to the widespread deployment of AEDs that can be used by lay responders in the community. AEDs are also available in hospitals for use by all staff, but manual defibrillators are appropriate for use by clinical staff only as part of ALS.

Strategies before defibrillation

Safe use of oxygen

In an oxygen-enriched atmosphere, sparking from poorly applied defibrillator paddles can cause a fire. Taking the following precautions can minimise the risk of fire during attempted defibrillation:

- Take off any oxygen mask or nasal cannulae and place them at least 1 m away from the patient's chest.
- Leave the ventilation bag connected to the tracheal tube or other airway adjunct. Alternatively, disconnect the ventilation bag from the tracheal tube and remove it at least 1 m from the patient's chest during defibrillation.
- Self-adhesive defibrillation pads may minimise the risk of sparks compared with manual paddles.

Chest hair

Rapid shaving of the area of intended electrode placement may be necessary, but do not delay defibrillation if a shaver is not immediately available.

Paddle force

If using paddles, apply them firmly to the chest wall, the optimal force being 8 kg in adults and 5 kg in children 1–8 y using adult paddles. Bare metal paddles require water-based gel pads placed between their metal face and the patient's skin. Gels and creams may smear between the paddles, risking arcing and ineffective defibrillation; their use is not recommended.

Electrode position

Placement for ventricular arrhythmias

The right (sternal) electrode is placed to the right of the sternum, below the clavicle. The apical paddle is placed in the mid-axillary line, approximately level with the V6 ECG electrode or female breast. This position should be clear of any breast tissue. It is important that this electrode is placed sufficiently laterally.

Other acceptable pad positions include:

- Each electrode placed on the lateral chest walls, one on the right and the other on the left side (bi-axillary).
- One electrode in the standard apical position and the other on the right or left upper back.
- One electrode anteriorly, over the left precordium, and the other electrode posteriorly to the heart, just inferior to the left scapula.

Placement for atrial arrhythmias

Anteroposterior electrode placement may be more effective than the traditional antero-apical position in cardioversion of atrial fibrillation. Either position is acceptable.

Implantable medical devices [e.g. permanent pacemaker, automatic implantable cardioverter defibrillator (AICD)] may be damaged during defibrillation if current is discharged through electrodes placed directly over the device. Place the electrode away from the device or use an alternative electrode position. Remove transdermal drug patches prior to defibrillation if they are placed on the chest wall.

Respiratory phase

Attempt defibrillation at end-expiration. Minimise positive end expiratory pressure (PEEP) during defibrillation.

Pads versus paddles

Self-adhesive defibrillation pads are safe and effective and are an acceptable alternative to standard defibrillation paddles. They enable the operator to defibrillate the patient from a safe distance rather than leaning over the patient, as occurs with paddles. When used for initial monitoring of a rhythm, both defibrillation pads and paddles provide more rapid delivery of the first shock compared with using standard ECG electrodes, but pads are quicker than paddles.

CPR versus defibrillation as the initial treatment

Although the previous guidelines have recommended immediate defibrillation for all shockable rhythms, recent evidence has suggested that a period of CPR before defibrillation may be beneficial after prolonged collapse. In clinical studies where response times exceeded 4–5 min, a period of 1.5–3 min of CPR by paramedics or EMS physicians before shock delivery improved survival to hospital discharge for adults with out-of-hospital VF or VT compared with immediate defibrillation. It may not be possible to extrapolate the outcomes achieved by paramedic-provided CPR, which includes intubation and delivery of 100% oxygen, to those that may be achieved by lay people providing relatively poor quality CPR with mouth-to-mouth ventilation.

It is reasonable for EMS personnel to give a period of about 2 min of CPR (i.e. about five cycles at 30:2) before defibrillation in patients with prolonged collapse (>5 min). The duration of collapse is frequently difficult to estimate accurately and it may be simplest if EMS personnel are instructed to provide this period of CPR before attempted defibrillation in any cardiac arrest they have not witnessed. Given the relatively weak evidence available, individual EMS directors should determine whether to implement a CPR before defibrillation strategy; inevitably, protocols will vary depending on the local circumstances.

Lay people and first responders using AEDS should deliver the shock as soon as possible.

There is no evidence to support or refute CPR before defibrillation for in-hospital cardiac arrest. We recommend shock delivery as soon as possible following in-hospital VF/VT cardiac arrest.

Delivery of defibrillation

One-shock versus three-shock sequence

With a three-shock protocol recommended in the 2000 guidelines, interruptions in CPR due to rhythm analysis by AEDs were significant. Delays of up to 37 s between delivery of shocks and recommencing chest compressions have been reported. With first shock efficacy of biphasic waveforms exceeding 90%, failure to cardiovert VF successfully is more likely to suggest the need for a period of CPR rather than a further shock. Thus, immediately after giving a single shock, and without reassessing the rhythm or feeling for a pulse, resume CPR (30 compressions:two ventilations) for 2 min before delivering another shock (if indicated). Even if the defibrillation attempt is successful in restoring a perfusing rhythm, it is very rare for a pulse to be palpable immediately after defibrillation and the delay in trying to palpate a pulse will further compromise the myocardium if a perfusing rhythm has not been restored. If a perfusing rhythm has been restored, giving chest compressions does not increase the chance of VF recurring. In the presence of post-shock asystole, chest compressions may induce VF.

This single shock strategy is applicable to both monophasic and biphasic defibrillators.

Waveforms and energy levels

First shock efficacy for long duration VF/ VT is greater with biphasic than monophasic waveforms and therefore use of the former is recommended whenever possible. Optimal energy levels for both monophasic (Figures 3.3 and 3.4) and biphasic waveforms (Figures 3.5 and 3.6) are unknown. The recommendations for energy levels are based on a consensus following careful review of the current literature.

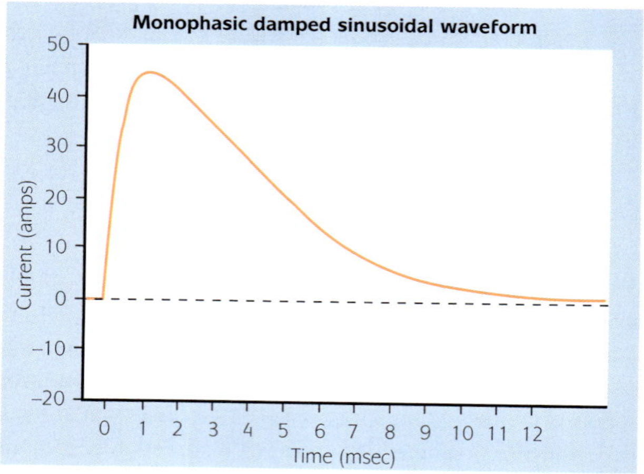

Figure 3.3. Monophasic damped sinusoidal waveform.

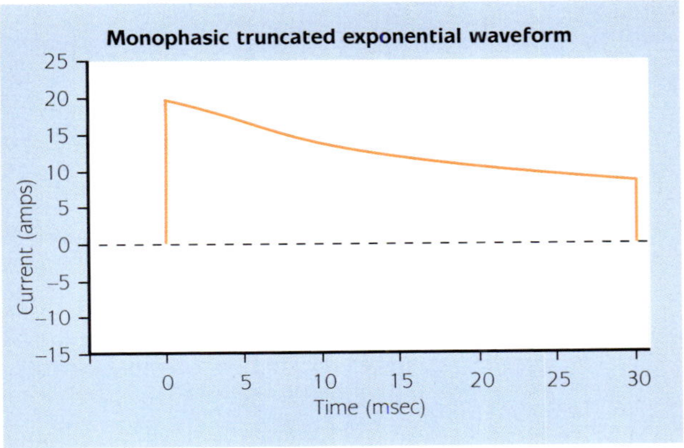

Figure 3.4. Monophasic truncated exponential waveform.

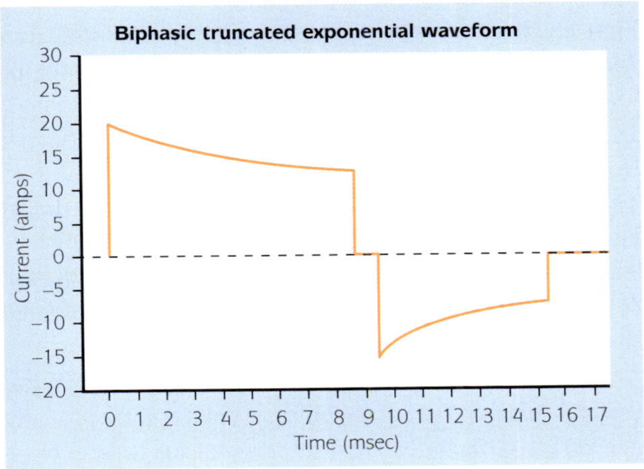

Figure 3.5. Biphasic truncated exponential waveform.

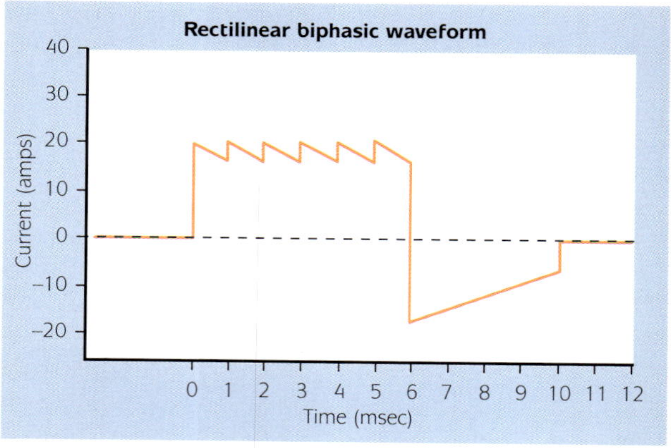

Figure 3.6. Rectilinear biphasic waveform.

First shock

Monophasic defibrillators Because of the lower efficacy of the monophasic waveform compared with a biphasic waveform, the recommended initial energy level for the first shock using a monophasic defibrillator is 360 J.

Biphasic defibrillators The initial biphasic shock should be no lower than 120 J for rectilinear biphasic (RLB) waveforms and 150 J for biphasic truncated exponential (BTE) waveforms. Ideally, the initial biphasic shock energy should be at least 150 J for all waveforms.

Manufacturers should display the effective waveform dose range on the face of the biphasic device. If the provider is unaware of the effective dose range of the device, use a dose of 200 J for the first shock. This 200 J default energy has been chosen because it falls within the reported range of selected doses that are effective for first and subsequent biphasic shocks and can be provided by every biphasic manual defibrillator available today. It is a consensus default dose and not a recommended ideal dose. If biphasic devices are clearly labelled and providers are familiar with the devices they use in clinical care, there will be no need for the default 200 J dose. Ongoing research is necessary to firmly establish the most appropriate initial settings for both monophasic and biphasic defibrillators.

Second and subsequent shocks

Monophasic defibrillators Because the initial shock has been unsuccessful at 360 J, give second and subsequent shocks at 360 J.

Biphasic defibrillators If the initial shock has been unsuccessful, it may be worth attempting the second and subsequent shocks with a higher energy level. However, there is no evidence to support either a fixed or escalating energy protocol. Both strategies are acceptable. If the provider is unaware of the effective dose range of the biphasic device and has used the default 200 J dose for the first shock, use either an equal or higher dose for second or subsequent shocks, depending on the capabilities of the device.

Airway management and ventilation

Patients requiring resuscitation often have an obstructed airway. Prompt assessment, with control of the airway and ventilation of the lungs, is essential. Without adequate oxygenation it may be impossible to restore a spontaneous cardiac output. In a witnessed cardiac arrest in the vicinity of a defibrillator, attempted defibrillation should take precedence over opening the airway.

Give high flow oxygen. Masks with non-rebreathing reservoir bags are more effective than standard masks for giving oxygen to the patient breathing spontaneously.

Basic airway manoeuvres

Assess the airway. Once any degree of obstruction is recognised, use one of the following manoeuvres to open the airway.

Head tilt and chin lift

The rescuer's hand is placed on the patient's forehead and the head gently tilted back; the fingertips of the other hand are placed under the point of the patient's chin, which is gently lifted to stretch the anterior neck structures.

Jaw thrust

The rescuer's index and other fingers are placed behind the angle of the mandible, and pressure is applied upwards and forwards. Using the thumbs, the mouth is opened slightly by downward displacement of the chin. This is the manoeuvre of choice for patients with suspected spinal cord injury.

Airway adjuncts

Simple airway adjuncts are often helpful, and sometimes essential, to maintain an open airway.

Oropharyngeal airway

An *estimate* of the size required is obtained by selecting an airway with a length corresponding to the vertical distance between the patient's incisors and the angle of the jaw. Insertion should be attempted only in comatose patients to avoid stimulating vomiting.

Nasopharyngeal airway

A nasopharyngeal airway is tolerated better than an oropharyngeal airway and may be life-saving in patients with clenched jaws, trismus or maxillofacial injuries, when insertion of an oral airway is impossible. Inadvertent insertion of a nasopharyngeal airway through a fracture of the skull base and into the cranial vault is extremely rare; death from airway obstruction is common. If an oropharyngeal airway cannot be inserted and the airway remains obstructed, gentle insertion of a nasopharyngeal airway may be life-saving. Using the patient's little finger or anterior nares to assess appropriate size is unreliable. Sizes of 6–7 mm are suitable for adults.

Ventilation

Artificial ventilation is started as soon as possible in any patient in whom spontaneous ventilation is inadequate or absent. Expired air ventilation (rescue breathing) is effective but the rescuer's expired oxygen concentration is only 16–17%, so it must be replaced as soon as possible by ventilation with oxygen-enriched air. The pocket resuscitation mask enables mouth-to-mask ventilation. Some enable supplemental oxygen to be given. Use a two-hand technique to maximise the seal with the patient's face.

Deliver each breath over approximately 1 s and give a volume that corresponds to normal chest movement; this represents a compromise between giving an adequate volume, minimising the risk of gastric inflation and allowing adequate time for chest compressions. During CPR with unprotected airway, two ventilations are delivered after each sequence of 30 chest compressions.

Self-inflating bag

The self-inflating bag can be connected to a face mask, tracheal tube or alternative airway device. If a reservoir system is attached and the oxygen flow is increased to approximately 10 l min^{-1}, an inspired oxygen concentration of 85% can be achieved.

The two-person technique for bag-mask ventilation is preferable. One person holds the face mask in place using a jaw thrust with both hands and an assistant squeezes the bag. In this way, a better seal can be achieved and the patient's lungs can be ventilated more effectively and safely.

Once an airway device has been inserted, ventilate the lungs at 10 breaths min^{-1} and continue chest compressions without pausing during ventilations.

Automatic ventilators

An automatic resuscitator should be set initially to deliver a tidal volume of 6–7 ml kg^{-1} at 10 breaths min^{-1}. Once the patient is intubated, use of the automatic resuscitator will enable the rescuer to undertake other tasks and, if set appropriately, will prevent hyperventilation.

Alternative airway devices

Laryngeal mask airway (LMA)

The laryngeal mask airway is relatively easy to insert and ventilation using the LMA is more efficient and easier than with a bag-valve-face mask. If gas leakage is excessive, chest compressions will have to be interrupted to enable ventilation. Pulmonary aspiration is rare when using the LMA during cardiac arrest.

The Combitube

The Combitube appears as safe and effective as tracheal intubation for airway management during cardiac arrest. Great care must be taken to avoid attempting to ventilate the lungs through the wrong port of the Combitube.

Tracheal intubation

There is insufficient evidence to support or refute the use of any specific technique to maintain an airway and provide ventilation in adults with cardiopulmonary arrest. Despite this, tracheal intubation is perceived as the optimal method of providing and maintaining a clear and secure airway. It should be used only when trained personnel are available to carry out the procedure with a high level of skill and confidence.

The perceived advantages of tracheal intubation over bag-mask ventilation include: maintenance of a patient airway, which is protected from aspiration of gastric contents or blood from the oropharynx; ability to provide an adequate tidal volume reliably even when chest compressions are uninterrupted; the potential to free the rescuer's hands for other tasks; the ability to suction airway secretions; and the provision of a route for giving drugs. Use of the bag-mask is more likely to cause gastric distension, which, theoretically, is more likely to cause regurgitation with risk of aspiration. However, there are no reliable data to indicate that the incidence of aspiration is any less in cardiac arrest patients ventilated with bag-mask versus those that are ventilated via tracheal tube.

The perceived disadvantages of tracheal intubation over bag-valve-mask ventilation include: the risk of an unrecognised misplaced tracheal tube, which in patients with out-of-hospital cardiac arrest ranges from 6% to 14%; a prolonged time without chest compressions while intubation is attempted; and a comparatively high failure rate. Intubation success rates correlate with the intubation experience attained by individual paramedics. Rates for failure to intubate are as high as 50% in pre-hospital systems with a low patient volume and providers who do not perform intubation frequently. The cost of training pre-hospital staff to undertake intubation should also be considered. Healthcare personnel who undertake pre-hospital intubation should do so only within a structured, monitored programme, which should include comprehensive competency-based training and regular opportunities to refresh skills.

Rescuers must weigh the risks and benefits of intubation against the need to provide effective chest compressions. The intubation attempt will require interruption of chest compressions but once an advanced airway is in place ventilation will not require interruption of chest compressions. Personnel skilled in advanced airway management should be able to undertake laryngoscopy without stopping chest compressions – a brief pause in chest compressions will be required as the tube is passed through the vocal cords. Alternatively, to avoid any interruptions in chest compressions, the intubation attempt may be deferred until return of spontaneous circulation. No intubation attempt should take longer than 30 s: if intubation has not been achieved after this time, recommence bag-mask ventilation. After intubation, tube placement must be confirmed and the tube secured adequately.

Confirmation of correct placement of the tracheal tube

Unrecognised oesophageal intubation is the most serious complication of attempted tracheal intubation – routine use of primary and secondary techniques to confirm correct placement of the tracheal tube should reduce this risk. Primary assessment includes observation of chest expansion bilaterally, auscultation over the lung fields bilaterally in the axillae (breath sounds should be equal and adequate) and over the epigastrium (breath sounds should not be heard). Clinical signs of correct tube placement (condensation in the tube, chest rise, breath sounds on auscultation of lungs and inability to hear gas entering the stomach) are not completely reliable. Secondary confirmation of tracheal tube placement by an exhaled CO_2 or oesophageal detection device should reduce the risk of unrecognised oesophageal intubation. If there is doubt about correct tube placement, use the laryngoscope and look directly to see if the tube passes through the vocal cords.

None of the secondary confirmation techniques will differentiate a tube placed in a main bronchus from one placed correctly in the trachea. There are inadequate data to identify the optimal method of confirming tube placement during cardiac arrest and all devices should be considered as adjuncts to other confirmatory techniques.

During cardiac arrest, pulmonary blood flow may be so low that there is insufficient exhaled CO_2, so the CO_2 detector does not identify a correctly placed tracheal tube. When exhaled CO_2 is detected in cardiac arrest, it indicates reliably that the tube is in the trachea or main bronchus, but when it is absent, tracheal tube placement is best confirmed with an oesophageal detector device. A variety of electronic as well as simple, inexpensive, colorimetric CO_2 detectors are available for both in-hospital and out-of-hospital use.

Cricothyroidotomy

If it is impossible to ventilate an apnoeic patient with a bag-mask, or to pass a tracheal tube or alternative airway device, delivery of oxygen through a needle or surgical cricothyroidotomy may be life-saving.

Peri-arrest arrhythmias

Cardiac arrhythmias are well recognised complications of myocardial infarction. They may precede VF or follow successful defibrillation. The treatment algorithms described in this section have been designed to enable the non-specialist advanced life support (ALS) provider to treat the patient effectively and safely in an emergency; for this reason, they have been kept as simple as possible. If patients are not acutely ill there may be several other treatment options, including the use of drugs (oral or parenteral) that will be less familiar to the non-expert. In this situation there will be time to seek advice from cardiologists or other senior doctors with the appropriate expertise.

More comprehensive information on the management of arrhythmias can be found at www.escardio.org.

Principles of treatment

In all cases, give oxygen and insert an intravenous cannula while the arrhythmia is assessed. Whenever possible, record a 12-lead ECG; this will help determine the precise rhythm, either before treatment or retrospectively, if necessary with the help of an expert. Correct any electrolyte abnormalities (e.g. K^+, Mg^{2+}, Ca^{2+}).

The assessment and treatment of all arrhythmias addresses two factors: the condition of the patient (stable versus unstable) and the nature of the arrhythmia.

Adverse signs

The presence or absence of adverse signs or symptoms will dictate the appropriate treatment for most arrhythmias. The following adverse factors indicate a patient who is unstable because of the arrhythmia.

Clinical evidence of low cardiac output

This is seen as pallor, sweating, cold, clammy extremities (increased sympathetic activity), impaired consciousness (reduced cerebral blood flow) and hypotension (e.g. systolic blood pressure <90 mmHg).

Excessive tachycardia

Coronary blood flow occurs predominantly during diastole. Very high heart rates (e.g. >150 min^{-1}) reduce diastole critically, decreasing coronary blood flow and causing myocardial ischaemia. Broad complex tachycardias are tolerated less well by the heart than narrow complex tachycardias.

Excessive bradycardia

This is defined as a heart rate of <40 beats min^{-1}, but rates of <60 beats min^{-1} may not be tolerated by patients with poor cardiac reserve. Even a higher heart rate may be inappropriately slow for a patient with a low stroke volume.

Heart failure

In reducing coronary artery blood flow, arrhythmias compromise myocardial performance. In acute situations this is manifested by pulmonary oedema (failure of the left ventricle), or raised jugular venous pressure, and hepatic engorgement (failure of the right ventricle).

Chest pain

The presence of chest pain implies that the arrhythmia (particularly a tachyarrhythmia) is causing myocardial ischaemia. This is especially important if there is underlying coronary artery disease or structural heart disease in which myocardial ischaemia is likely to lead to further life-threatening complications including cardiac arrest.

Treatment options

Having determined the rhythm and the presence or absence of adverse signs, there are broadly three options for immediate treatment:

1. Anti-arrhythmic (and other) drugs.
2. Attempted electrical cardioversion.
3. Cardiac pacing.

All anti-arrhythmic treatments – physical manoeuvres, drugs or electrical treatment – can also be pro-arrhythmic, so that clinical deterioration may be caused by the treatment rather than lack of effect. Furthermore, the use of multiple anti-arrhythmic drugs or high doses of a single drug can cause myocardial depression and hypotension. This may cause a deterioration of the cardiac rhythm.

Anti-arrhythmic drugs are slower in effect and less reliable than electrical cardioversion in converting a tachycardia to sinus rhythm; thus, drugs tend to be reserved for stable patients without adverse signs and electrical cardioversion is usually the preferred treatment for the unstable patient displaying adverse signs.

Once the arrhythmia has been treated successfully repeat the 12-lead ECG to enable detection of any underlying abnormalities that may require long-term therapy.

Bradycardia

A bradycardia is defined strictly as a heart rate of <60 beats min^{-1}. However, it is more helpful to classify a bradycardia as absolute (<40 beats min^{-1}) or relative, when the heart rate is inappropriately slow for the haemodynamic state of the patient.

The first step in the assessment of bradycardia is to determine if the patient is unstable (Figure 3.7). The following adverse signs may indicate instability:

- Systolic blood pressure <90 mmHg.
- Heart rate <40 beats min^{-1}.
- Ventricular arrhythmias requiring suppression.
- Heart failure.

If adverse signs are present, give atropine 500 mcg intravenously and, if necessary, repeat every 3–5 min, to a total of 3 mg. Paradoxically, doses of atropine of less than 500 mcg may cause further slowing of the heart rate. In healthy volunteers a dose of 3 mg produces the maximum achievable increase in resting heart rate. Use atropine cautiously in the presence of acute coronary ischaemia or myocardial infarction; increased heart rate may worsen ischaemia or increase the zone of infarction.

If a satisfactory response is achieved with atropine, or if the patient is stable, next determine the risk of asystole, which is indicated by:

- Recent asystole.
- Möbitz type II AV block.
- Complete (third degree) heart block (especially with broad QRS or initial heart rate less than 40 min^{-1}).
- Ventricular standstill of more than 3 s.

Pacing is likely to be required if there is a risk of asystole,

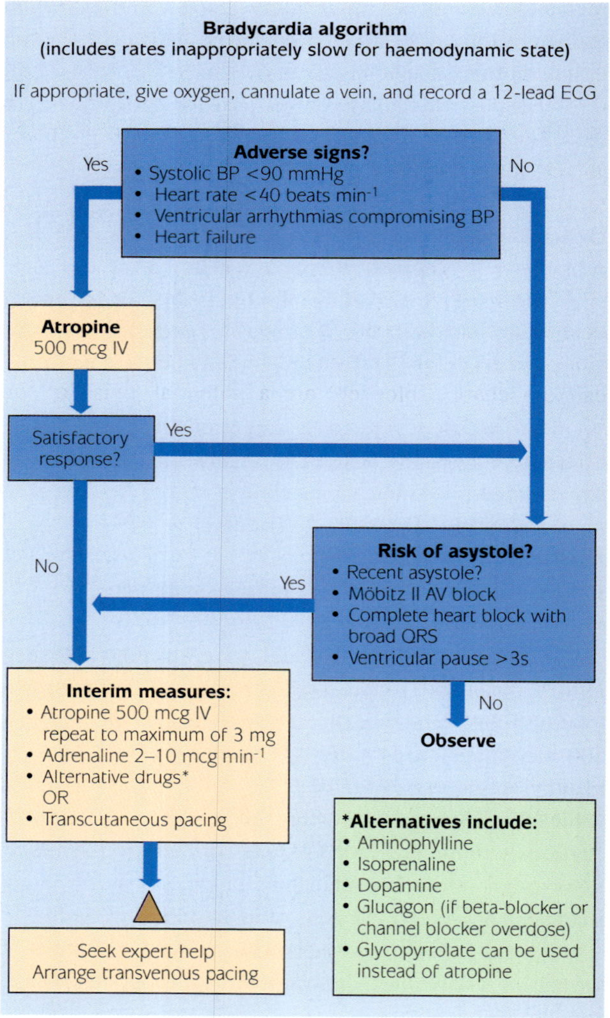

Figure 3.7. Bradycardia algorithm.

or if the patient is unstable and has failed to respond satisfactorily to atropine. Under these circumstances, the definitive treatment is transvenous pacing. One or more of the following interventions can be used to improve the patient's condition while waiting for the appropriate personnel and facilities:

- Transcutaneous pacing.
- Adrenaline infusion in the range of 2–10 mcg min^{-1} titrated to response.

Other drugs that can be given for symptomatic bradycardia include: dopamine, isoprenaline and theophylline. Consider giving intravenous glucagon if beta-blockers or calcium channel-blockers are a potential cause of the bradycardia. Do not give atropine to patients with cardiac transplants – paradoxically it can cause a high degree AV block or even sinus arrest.

Complete heart block with a narrow QRS is not an absolute indication for pacing because atrioventricular junctional ectopic pacemakers (with a narrow QRS) may provide a reasonable and stable heart rate.

Pacing

Transcutaneous pacing

Initiate transcutaneous pacing immediately if there is no response to atropine, if atropine is unlikely to be effective, or if the patient is severely symptomatic, particularly if there is high degree block (Möbitz type II 2° block or 3° block). Transcutaneous pacing can be painful and may fail to produce effective mechanical capture. Verify mechanical capture and reassess the patient's condition. Use analgesia and sedation to control pain, and attempt to identify the cause of the bradyarrhythmia.

Fist pacing

If atropine is ineffective, and transcutaneous pacing is not immediately available, fist pacing can be attempted while waiting for pacing equipment: give serial rhythmic blows with the closed fist over the left lower edge of the sternum to pace the heart at a physiological rate of 50–70 beats min^{-1}.

Tachycardias

In the peri-arrest setting, many treatment principles are common to all the tachycardias. For this reason, they have been combined into a single tachycardia algorithm (Figure 3.8).

If the patient is unstable and deteriorating with signs and symptoms caused by the tachycardia (e.g. impaired conscious level, chest pain, heart failure, hypotension or other signs of shock), attempt synchronised cardioversion immediately. In patients with otherwise normal hearts, serious signs and symptoms are uncommon if the ventricular rate is <150 min^{-1}. Patients with impaired cardiac function or significant comorbidity may be symptomatic and unstable at lower heart rates. If cardioversion fails to restore sinus rhythm and the patient remains unstable, give amiodarone 300 mg intravenously over 10–20 min and reattempt electrical cardioversion. The loading dose of amiodarone can be followed by an infusion of 900 mg over 24 h.

Serial DC shocks are not appropriate for recurrent (within hours or days) paroxysms (self-terminating episodes) of atrial fibrillation. This is relatively common in critically ill patients who may have ongoing precipitating factors causing the arrhythmia (e.g. metabolic disturbance, sepsis). Cardioversion does not prevent subsequent arrhythmias. If there are recurrent episodes, treat them with drugs.

Synchronised electrical cardioversion

If electrical cardioversion is used to convert atrial or ventricular tachyarrhythmias, the shock must be synchronised with the R wave of the ECG rather than with the T wave. By avoiding the relative refractory period in this way, the risk of inducing ventricular fibrillation is minimised. Conscious patients must be anaesthetised or sedated before synchronised cardioversion is attempted. For a broad complex tachycardia and atrial fibrillation, start with 200 J monophasic or 120–150 J biphasic, and increase in increments if this fails. Atrial flutter and paroxysmal supraventricular tachycardia (SVT) will often convert with lower energies: start with 100 J monophasic or 70–120 J biphasic.

If the patient with tachycardia is stable (no serious signs or symptoms caused by the tachycardia) and is not deteriorating, there is time to evaluate the rhythm using the 12-lead ECG and determine treatment options. The ALS provider may not have the expertise to diagnose the tachycardia precisely but should be capable of differentiating between sinus tachycardia, narrow complex supraventricular tachycardia (SVT) and wide complex tachycardia. If the patient is stable there is normally time to consult an expert. If the patient becomes unstable proceed immediately to synchronised electrical cardioversion. Management of patients with significant comorbid conditions and symptomatic tachycardia requires treatment of the comorbid conditions.

Broad complex tachycardia

In broad complex tachycardias the QRS complexes are >0.12 s and are usually ventricular in origin. Although broad complex tachycardias may be caused by supraventricular rhythms with aberrant conduction, in the unstable patient in the peri-arrest context, assume they are ventricular in origin. In the stable patient with broad complex tachycardia, the next step is to determine if the rhythm is regular or irregular.

Regular broad complex tachycardia

A regular broad complex tachycardia is likely to be VT or SVT with bundle branch block. Stable VT can be treated with amiodarone 300 mg intravenously over 20–60 min followed by an infusion of 900 mg over 24 h. If the broad complex regular tachycardia is thought to be SVT with bundle branch block, give adenosine using the strategy indicated for narrow complex tachycardia (below).

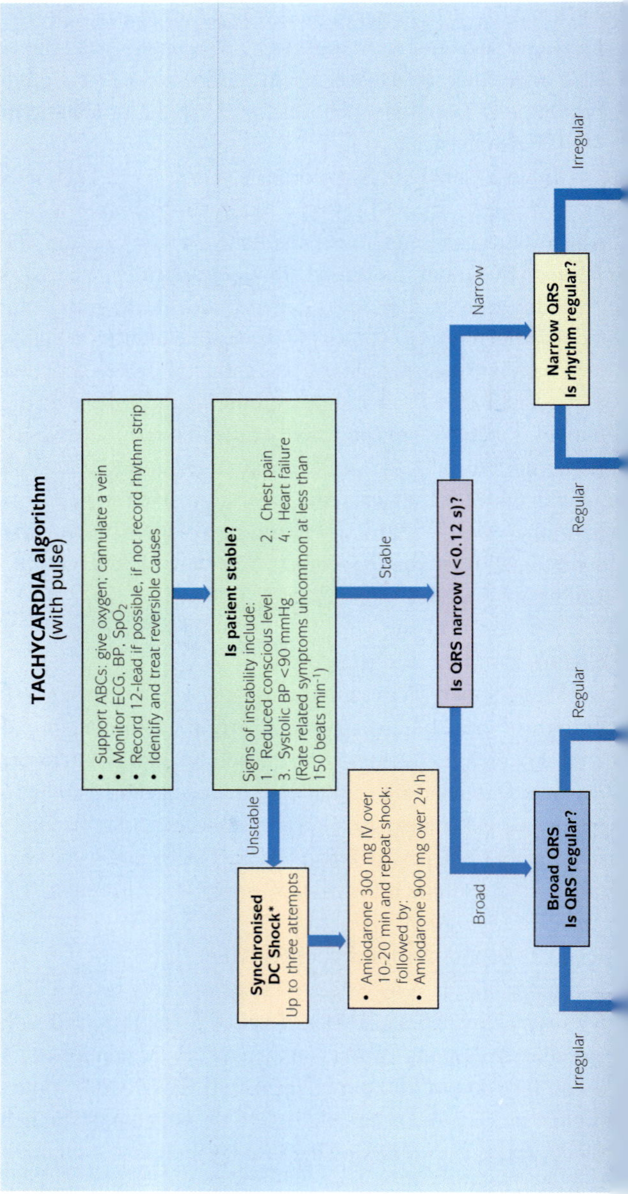

Figure 3.8. Tachycardia algorithm.

Seek expert help

Possibilities include:
- **AF with bundle branch block** treat as for narrow complex
- **Pre-excited AF** consider amiodarone
- **Polymorphic VT** (e.g. torsades de pointes – give magnesium 2 g over 10 min)

If **Ventricular Tachycardia** (or uncertain rhythm)
- Amiodarone 300 mg IV over 20-60 min; then 900 mg over 24 h

If previously confirmed **SVT with bundle branch block**:
- Give adenosine as for regular narrow complex tachycardia

- Use vagal manoeuvres
- Adenosine 6 mg rapid IV bolus; if unsuccessful give 12 mg; if unsuccessful give further 12 mg.
- Monitor ECG continuously

Normal sinus rhythm restored?

Yes:

Probable **re-entry PSVT:**
- Record 12-lead ECG in sinus rhythm
- If recurs, give adenosine again and consider choice of anti-arrhythmic prophylaxis

No:

Seek expert help

Possible **atrial flutter**
- Control rate (e.g. beta-blocker)

Irregular narrow complex tachycardia

Probable **atrial fibrillation**

Control rate with:
- Beta-blocker IV, digoxin IV or dilitiazem IV

If onset <48 h consider:
- Amiodarone 300 mg IV 20–60 min; then 900 mg over 24 h

*Attempted electrical cardioversion is always undertaken under sedation or general anaesthesia

Irregular broad complex tachycardia

This is most likely to be atrial fibrillation (AF) with bundle branch block, but careful examination of a 12-lead ECG (if necessary by an expert) may enable confident identification of the rhythm. Another possible cause is AF with ventricular pre-excitation [in patients with Wolff–Parkinson–White (WPW) syndrome]. There is more variation in the appearance and width of the QRS complexes than in AF with bundle branch block. A third possible cause is polymorphic VT (e.g. torsades de pointes), but polymorphic VT is unlikely to be present without adverse features.

Seek expert help with the assessment and treatment of irregular broad complex tachyarrhythmia. If treating AF with bundle branch block, treat as for AF (see below). If pre-excited AF (or atrial flutter) is suspected avoid adenosine, digoxin, verapamil and diltiazem. These drugs block the AV node and cause a relative increase in pre-excitation. Electrical cardioversion is usually the safest treatment option.

Treat torsades de pointes VT immediately by stopping all drugs known to prolong QT interval. Correct electrolyte abnormalities, especially hypokalaemia. Give magnesium sulphate 2 g intravenously over 10 min. Obtain expert help as other treatment (e.g. overdrive pacing) may be indicated to prevent relapse once the arrhythmia has been corrected. If adverse features develop (usual) arrange immediate synchronised cardioversion. If the patient becomes pulseless, attempt defibrillation immediately (cardiac arrest algorithm).

Narrow complex tachycardia

Regular narrow complex tachycardias include:

- Sinus tachycardia.
- AV nodal re-entry tachycardia – AVNRT (the commonest type of SVT).
- AV re-entry tachycardia – AVRT (due to WPW syndrome).
- Atrial flutter with regular AV conduction (usually 2:1).

Irregular narrow complex tachycardia is most commonly atrial fibrillation (AF) or sometimes atrial flutter with variable AV conduction ('variable block').

Regular narrow complex tachycardia

Sinus tachycardia This is a common physiological response to a stimulus such as exercise or anxiety. In a sick patient it may be seen in response to many stimuli such as pain, fever, anaemia, blood loss and heart failure. Treatment is almost always directed at the underlying cause – trying to slow sinus tachycardia that has occurred in response to most of these situations will make the situation worse.

AVNRT and AVRT (paroxysmal SVT) AV nodal re-entry tachycardia is the commonest type of paroxysmal SVT, often seen in people without any other form of heart disease and is relatively uncommon in a peri-arrest setting. It causes a regular narrow complex tachycardia, often with no clearly visible atrial activity on the ECG, with heart rates usually well above the typical range of sinus rates at rest (60–120 min^{-1}). It is usually benign, unless there is additional co-incidental structural heart disease or coronary disease, but may cause symptoms that the patient finds frightening.

AV re-entry tachycardia is seen in patients with the WPW syndrome and is also usually benign unless there happens to be additional structural heart disease. The common type of AVRT is a regular narrow complex tachycardia, also often having no visible atrial activity on the ECG.

Atrial flutter with regular AV conduction (often 2:1 block) This produces a regular narrow complex tachycardia in which it may be difficult to see atrial activity and identify flutter waves with confidence, so may be indistinguishable initially from AVNRT and AVRT.

When atrial flutter with 2:1 block or even 1:1 conduction is accompanied by bundle branch block it produces a regular broad complex tachycardia that will usually be very difficult to distinguish from VT; treatment of this rhythm as if it were VT will usually be effective or will lead to slowing of the ventricular response and identification of the rhythm.

Most typical atrial flutter has an atrial rate of about 300 min^{-1}, so atrial flutter with 2:1 block tends to produce a tachycardia of about 150 min^{-1}. Much faster rates (170 min^{-1} or more) are unlikely to be due to atrial flutter with 2:1 block.

Treatment of regular narrow complex tachycardia If the patient is unstable with adverse features caused by the arrhythmia, attempt synchronised electrical cardioversion. It is reasonable to give adenosine to an unstable patient with a regular narrow complex tachycardia while preparations are made for synchronised cardioversion; however, do not delay electrical cardioversion if the adenosine fails to restore sinus rhythm.

In the absence of adverse features:

- Start with vagal manoeuvres. Carotid sinus massage or the Valsalva manoeuvre will terminate up to a quarter of episodes of paroxysmal SVT. A Valsalva manoeuvre (forced expiration against a closed glottis) in the supine position may be the most effective technique. Avoid carotid massage if a carotid bruit is present; rupture of an atheromatous plaque could cause cerebral embolism and stroke. In the context of acute ischaemia or digitalis toxicity, sudden bradycardia may trigger ventricular fibrillation. Record an ECG (preferably multilead) during each manoeuvre. If the rhythm is atrial flutter, slowing of the ventricular response will often occur and demonstrate flutter waves.
- If the arrhythmia persists and is not atrial flutter, use adenosine. Give 6 mg as a rapid intravenous bolus. Record an ECG (preferably multilead) during each injection. If the ventricular rate slows transiently, but the arrhythmia then persists, look for atrial activity such as atrial flutter or other atrial tachycardia and treat accordingly. If there is no response to adenosine 6 mg give a 12 mg bolus. If there is no response give one further 12 mg bolus.
- Successful termination of a tachyarrhythmia by vagal manoeuvres or adenosine indicates that it was almost

certainly AVNRT or AVRT. Monitor the patient for further rhythm abnormalities. Treat recurrence either with further adenosine or with a longer-acting drug with AV nodal blocking action (e.g. diltiazem or beta-blocker).

- Vagal manoeuvres or adenosine will terminate almost all AVNRT or AVRT within seconds. Failure to terminate a regular narrow complex tachycardia with adenosine suggests an atrial tachycardia such as atrial flutter.
- If adenosine is contraindicated or fails to terminate a regular narrow complex tachycardia without demonstrating that it is atrial flutter, give a calcium channel-blocker (e.g. verapamil 2.5–5 mg intravenously over 2 min).

Irregular narrow complex tachycardia

An irregular narrow complex tachycardia is most likely to be AF with an uncontrolled ventricular response or less commonly atrial flutter with variable AV block. Record a 12-lead ECG to identify the rhythm. If the patient is unstable with adverse features caused by the arrhythmia, attempt synchronised electrical cardioversion.

If there are no adverse features, treatment options include:

- Rate control by drug therapy.
- Rhythm control using drugs to encourage chemical cardioversion.
- Rhythm control by electrical cardioversion.
- Treatment to prevent complications (e.g. anticoagulation).

Obtain expert help to determine the most appropriate treatment for the individual patient. The longer a patient remains in AF the greater is the likelihood of atrial clot developing. In general, patients who have been in AF for more than 48 h should not be treated by cardioversion (electrical or chemical) until they have been fully anticoagulated or unless absence of atrial clot has been shown by trans-oesophageal echocardiography.

If the aim is to control heart rate, options include a beta-blocker, digoxin, diltiazem, magnesium, or combinations of these.

If the duration of AF is less than 48 h and rhythm control is considered appropriate, this may be attempted using amiodarone (300 mg intravenously over 20–60 min followed by 900 mg over 24 h). Ibutilide or flecainide can also be given for rhythm control, but expert advice should be obtained before using these drugs for this purpose. Electrical cardioversion remains an option in this setting and will restore sinus rhythm in more patients than chemical cardioversion.

Seek expert help if any patient with AF is known or found to have ventricular pre-excitation (WPW syndrome). Avoid giving adenosine, diltiazem, verapamil or digoxin to patients with pre-excited AF or atrial flutter as these drugs block the AV node and cause a relative increase in pre-excitation.

Post-resuscitation care

Return of spontaneous circulation (ROSC) is just the first step toward the goal of complete recovery from cardiac arrest. Interventions in the post-resuscitation period are likely to influence the final outcome significantly, yet there are relatively few data relating to this phase. Of 22,105 patients admitted to intensive care units in the UK after cardiac arrest, 9974 (45%) survived to leave intensive care and 6353 (30%) survived to hospital discharge [data from Intensive Care National Audit and Research Centre (ICNARC), London, December 1995–October 2004]. To return the patient to a state of normal cerebral function with no neurological deficit, a stable cardiac rhythm and normal haemodynamic function requires further resuscitation tailored to each patient's individual needs. The post-resuscitation phase starts at the location where ROSC is achieved, but once stabilised, the patient is transferred to the most appropriate high care area (e.g. intensive care unit, coronary care unit) for continued monitoring and treatment.

Airway and breathing

Patients who have had a brief period of cardiac arrest, having responded immediately to appropriate treatment, may achieve an immediate return of normal cerebral function. These patients do not require tracheal intubation and ventilation, but should be given oxygen via a face mask. Hypoxia and hypercarbia both increase the likelihood of a further cardiac arrest and may contribute to secondary brain injury. Consider tracheal intubation, sedation and controlled ventilation in any patient with obtunded cerebral function. Ensure the tracheal tube is positioned correctly well above the carina. Hypocarbia causes cerebral vasoconstriction and a decreased cerebral blood flow. After cardiac arrest, hypocapnoea induced by hyperventilation causes cerebral ischaemia. Adjust ventilation to achieve normocarbia and monitor this using the end-tidal CO_2 and arterial blood gas values. Adjust the inspired oxygen concentrations to achieve adequate arterial oxygen saturation.

Insert a gastric tube to decompress the stomach; gastric distension caused by mouth-to-mouth or bag-mask-valve ventilation will splint the diaphragm and impair ventilation. Avoid coughing – this will increase intracranial pressure and may cause transient hypoxaemia. Give adequate doses of sedative and, if absolutely necessary, give a neuromuscular-blocking drug. Obtain a chest radiograph to check the position of the tracheal tube and central venous lines etc., assess for pulmonary oedema, and to detect complications from CPR such as a pneumothorax associated with rib fractures.

Circulation

If there is evidence of coronary occlusion, consider the need for immediate revascularisation by thrombolysis or percutaneous coronary intervention (see acute coronary syndromes, page 87).

Haemodynamic instability is common after cardiac arrest and manifests as hypotension, low cardiac index and arrhythmias. This post-resuscitation myocardial dysfunction (or myocardial stunning) is usually transient and often reverses within 24–48 h. The post-resuscitation period is associated with marked elevations in plasma cytokine concentrations, which manifests as a sepsis-like syndrome and multiple organ dysfunction.

Infusion of fluids may be required to increase right heart filling pressures or, conversely, diuretics and vasodilators may be needed to treat left ventricular failure. In the ICU an arterial line for continuous blood pressure monitoring is essential and the use of a non-invasive or invasive (pulmonary artery catheter) cardiac output monitor may be helpful. Target the mean arterial blood pressure to achieve an adequate urine output, taking into consideration the patient's normal blood pressure.

Immediately after a cardiac arrest there is typically a period of hyperkalaemia. Subsequent endogenous catecholamine release promotes intracellular transportation of potassium, causing hypokalaemia. Hypokalaemia may predispose to ventricular arrhythmias. Give potassium to maintain the serum potassium concentration between 4.0 and 4.5 mmol l^{-1}.

Disability (optimising neurological recovery)

Cerebral perfusion

Immediately after ROSC there is a period of cerebral hyperaemia. After 15–30 min of reperfusion, however, global cerebral blood flow decreases and there is generalised hypoperfusion. Normal cerebral autoregulation is lost, leaving cerebral perfusion dependent on mean arterial pressure. Under these circumstances, hypotension will compromise cerebral blood flow severely and will compound any neurological injury. Thus, after ROSC, maintain mean arterial pressure at the patient's normal level.

Sedation

Although it has been common practice to sedate and ventilate patients for up to 24 h after ROSC, there are no data to support a defined period of ventilation, sedation and neuromuscular blockade after cardiac arrest. The duration of sedation and ventilation may be influenced by the use of therapeutic hypothermia (see below). There are no data to indicate whether or not the choice of sedation influences outcome, but short-acting drugs (e.g. propofol, alfentanil, remifentanil) will enable earlier neurological assessment.

Control of seizures

Seizures and/or myoclonus occur in 5–15% of adult patients who achieve ROSC, and in approximately 40% of those who remain comatose. Seizures increase cerebral metabolism by up to four-fold. Prolonged seizure activity may cause cerebral injury, and should be controlled with benzodiazepines, phenytoin, propofol, or a barbiturate. Each of these drugs can cause hypotension and this must be treated appropriately. Seizures and myoclonus per se are not related significantly to outcome, but status epilepticus and, in particular, status myoclonus are associated with a poor outcome.

Temperature control

Treatment of hyperpyrexia

A period of hyperthermia is common in the first 48 h after cardiac arrest. The risk of a poor neurological outcome increases for each degree of body temperature >37°C. Treat any hyperthermia occurring in the first 72 h after cardiac arrest with antipyretics or active cooling.

Therapeutic hypothermia

Mild hypothermia is thought to suppress many of the chemical reactions associated with reperfusion injury. These reactions include free radical production, excitatory amino acid release and calcium shifts, which can in turn lead to mitochondrial damage and apoptosis (programmed cell death). Two randomised clinical trials showed improved outcome in adults remaining comatose after initial resuscitation from out-of-hospital VF cardiac arrest, who were cooled within minutes to hours after ROSC.

Unconscious adult patients with spontaneous circulation after out-of-hospital VF cardiac arrest should be cooled to 32–34°C. Cooling should be started as soon as possible and continued for at least 12–24 h. Induced hypothermia might also benefit unconscious adult patients with spontaneous circulation after out-of-hospital cardiac arrest from a non-shockable rhythm, or cardiac arrest in hospital. Treat shivering by ensuring adequate sedation and giving neuromuscular-blocking drugs. Bolus doses of neuromuscular blockers are usually adequate but infusions are necessary occasionally. Re-warm the patient slowly (0.25–0.5°C h^{-1}) and avoid hyperthermia. The optimum target temperature, rate of cooling, duration of hypothermia and rate of re-warming have yet to be determined; further studies are essential.

External and/or internal cooling techniques can be used to initiate cooling. An infusion of 30 ml kg^{-1} of 4°C saline decreases core temperature by 1.5°C. Intravascular cooling enables more precise control of core temperature than external methods but it is unknown whether this improves outcome.

Complications of mild therapeutic hypothermia include increased infection, cardiovascular instability, coagulopathy, hyperglycaemia, and electrolyte abnormalities such as hypophosphataemia and hypomagnesaemia.

Other supportive therapies

Blood glucose control

There is a strong association between high blood glucose after resuscitation from cardiac arrest and poor neurological outcome. Persistent hyperglycaemia after stroke is associated with a worse neurological outcome. Tight control of blood glucose (4.4–6.1 mmol l^{-1} or 80–110 mg dl^{-1}) using insulin reduces hospital mortality in critically ill adults, but this has not been demonstrated in post-cardiac arrest patients specifically.

The optimal blood glucose target in critically ill patients has not been determined. Comatose patients are at particular risk from unrecognised hypoglycaemia and the risk of this complication occurring increases as the target blood glucose concentration is lowered.

In common with all critically ill patients, patients admitted to a critical care environment after cardiac arrest should have their blood glucose monitored frequently and hyperglycaemia treated with an insulin infusion. The blood glucose concentration that triggers insulin therapy and the target range of blood glucose concentrations should be determined by local policy. There is a need for studies of glucose control after cardiac arrest.

Prognostication

Once a heart has been resuscitated to a stable rhythm and cardiac output, the organ that influences an individual's survival most significantly is the brain. Two-thirds of those dying after admission to ICU following out-of-hospital cardiac arrest die from neurological injury. A quarter of those dying after admission to ICU following in-hospital cardiac arrest die from neurological injury. A means of predicting neurological outcome that can be applied to individual patients immediately after ROSC is required. Such a test of prognosis must have 100% specificity.

Clinical tests

There are no neurological signs that can predict outcome in the early hours after ROSC. By 3 d after the onset of coma relating to cardiac arrest, 50% of patients with no chance of ultimate recovery have died. In the remaining patients, the absence of pupil light reflexes on day 3 and an absent motor response to pain on day 3 are both independently predictive of a poor outcome (death or vegetative state) with very high specificity.

Biochemical tests

Measurement of serum neuron specific enolase (NSE) and protein S-100b may be useful in determining the outcome of a cardiac arrest, but until further research is undertaken these biochemical tests remain unreliable for predicting outcome in individual cases.

Electrophysiological tests

Median nerve somatosensory evoked potentials in normothermic patients, comatose for at least 72 h after cardiac arrest, predict poor outcome with 100% specificity. When recorded at least 24–48 h after ROSC, the electroencephalogram (EEG) provides limited prognostic information. A normal or grossly abnormal EEG predicts outcome reliably, but an EEG between these extremes is unreliable for prognostication.

Further reading

1. International Liaison Committee on Resuscitation. 2005 International Consensus on Cardiopulmonary Resuscitation and Emergency Cardiovascular Care Science with Treatment Recommendations. Resuscitation 2005;67:203–47.
2. European Resuscitation Council. European Resuscitation Council guidelines for resuscitation 2005. Resuscitation 2005;67(Suppl 1):S25–37, S39–86.

Chapter 4
Initial management of acute coronary syndromes

Hans-Richard Arntz, Leo Bossaert and Gerasimos Filippatos

Introduction

The incidence of acute myocardial infarction (AMI) is decreasing in many European countries. Although in-hospital mortality from AMI has been reduced significantly by modern reperfusion therapy and improved secondary prophylaxis, the overall 28-d mortality is virtually unchanged because about two-thirds of those that die do so before arrival at hospital. Thus, the best chance of improving survival after AMI is by improving treatment in the early, and particularly the out-of-hospital, phase of the disease.

The term acute coronary syndrome (ACS) encompasses three different entities of the acute manifestation of coronary heart disease: ST elevation myocardial infarction (STEMI), non-ST elevation myocardial infarction (NSTEMI) and unstable angina pectoris (UAP) (Figure 4.1). The common pathophysiology of ACS is a ruptured or eroded atherosclerotic plaque. Electrocardiographic (ECG) characteristics (absence or presence of ST elevation) differentiate STEMI from the other forms of ACS. An NSTEMI or UAP may present with ST segment depression or non-specific ST segment wave abnormalities, or even a normal ECG. In the absence of ST elevation, an increase in the plasma concentration of cardiac markers, particularly troponin T or I as the most specific markers of myocardial cell necrosis, indicates NSTEMI.

Acute coronary syndromes are the commonest cause of malignant arrhythmias leading to sudden cardiac death. The therapeutic goals are to treat acute life-threatening conditions, such as ventricular fibrillation (VF) or extreme bradycardias,

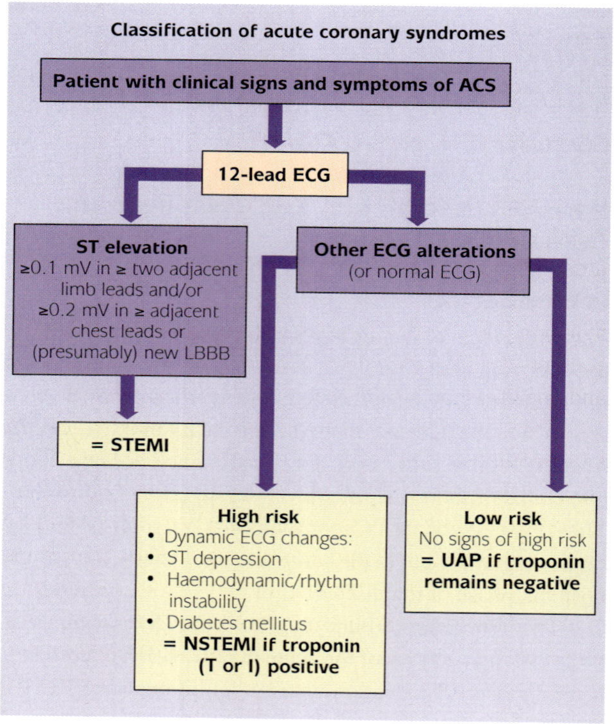

Figure 4.1. Classification of acute coronary syndromes.

and to preserve left ventricular function and prevent heart failure by minimising the extent of any myocardial infarction. These guidelines address the first hours after onset of symptoms. Out-of-hospital treatment and initial therapy in the emergency department may vary according to local capabilities, resources and regulations. The data supporting out-of-hospital treatment are usually extrapolated from studies of initial treatment early after hospital admission; there are only few high quality out-of-hospital studies. Comprehensive guidelines for the diagnosis and treatment of ACS with and without ST elevation have been published by the European Society of Cardiology and the American College of Cardiology/American Heart Association. The current recommendations are in line with these guidelines.

Diagnostic tests in acute coronary syndromes

Since early treatment offers the greatest benefits and myocardial ischaemia is the leading precipitant of sudden cardiac death, it is essential that the public are aware of the typical symptoms associated with ACS. Patients at risk, and their families, should be able to recognise characteristic symptoms such as chest pain, which may radiate into other areas of the upper body, often accompanied by other symptoms like dyspnoea, sweating, nausea or vomiting and syncope. They should understand the importance of early activation of the emergency medical service (EMS) system and, ideally, should be trained in basic life support (BLS).

EMS dispatchers must be trained to recognise ACS symptoms and to ask targeted questions. When an ACS is suspected, an EMS crew trained in advanced life support (ALS) and capable of making the diagnosis and starting treatment should be alerted. The sensitivity, specificity and clinical impact of various diagnostic strategies have been evaluated for ACS/AMI. These include signs and symptoms, the 12-lead ECG and biochemical markers of cardiac risk.

Signs and symptoms of ACS/AMI

Even though typical symptoms like radiating chest pain, shortness of breath or sweating may be more intense and generally last longer in patients with AMI, they are not adequately specific for a reliable diagnosis of AMI. A 12-lead ECG, cardiac biomarkers and other diagnostic tests are required before ACS or AMI can be ruled out in the presence of a typical history. Atypical symptoms or unusual presentations may occur in the elderly, in females, and in diabetics.

12-Lead ECG

A 12-lead ECG is the key investigation for assessment of an ACS. In the case of STEMI, it indicates the need for immediate reperfusion therapy [e.g. primary percutaneous coronary intervention (PCI) or pre-hospital thrombolysis]. Recording of a 12-lead ECG out-of-hospital enables advanced notification to the receiving facility and expedites treatment decisions after hospital arrival: in many studies, the time from hospital admission to initiating reperfusion therapy is reduced by 10 to 60 min. Recording and transmission of diagnostic quality ECGs to the hospital usually takes less than 5 min. Trained EMS personnel (emergency physicians, paramedics and nurses) can identify STEMI, defined by ST elevation of ≥0.1 mV elevation in at least two adjacent limb leads or >0.2 mV in two adjacent precordial leads, with a high specificity and sensitivity comparable to diagnostic accuracy in the hospital.

Biomarkers

In the presence of a suggestive history, the absence of ST elevation on the ECG and elevated concentrations of biomarkers (troponin T and troponin I, CK, CK-MB, myoglobin) characterise non-STEMI and distinguish it from STEMI and unstable angina, respectively. Elevated concentrations of troponin are particularly helpful in identifying patients at increased risk of adverse outcome. However, the delay in release of biomarkers from damaged myocardium prevents their use in diagnosing myocardial infarction in the first 4–6 h after the onset of symptoms.

Principles of acute treatment for ACS

Figure 4.2 schematically represents early treatment options for patients with signs and symptoms of acute coronary syndrome.

Nitrates

Glyceryl trinitrate is an effective treatment for ischaemic chest pain and has beneficial haemodynamic effects, e.g. dilation of the venous capacitance vessels, dilation of the coronary arteries and, to a minor degree, the peripheral arteries. Glyceryl trinitrate may be considered if the systolic blood pressure is higher than 90 mmHg and the patient has ongoing ischaemic chest pain. Glyceryl trinitrate can be useful in the treatment of acute pulmonary congestion. Do not use nitrates in patients with hypotension (systolic blood pressure

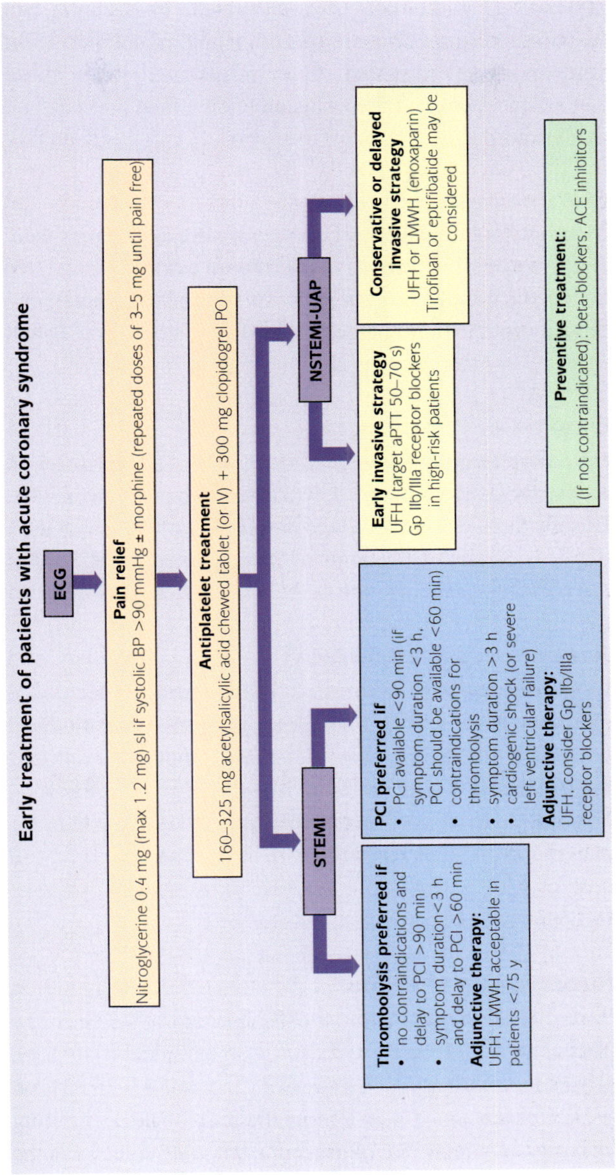

Figure 4.2. Early treatment of patients with acute coronary syndrome.

≤90 mmHg), particularly if combined with bradycardia, and in patients with inferior infarction and suspected right ventricular involvement. Use of nitrates under these circumstances may cause a sudden fall in blood pressure and cardiac output.

Morphine

Morphine is the analgesic of choice for nitrate-refractory pain. Being a dilator of venous capacitance vessels, it may have additional benefit in patients with pulmonary congestion. Give morphine in initial doses of 3–5 mg intravenously and repeat every few minutes until the patient is pain-free.

Oxygen

Give supplementary oxygen (4–8 l min^{-1}) to all patients with arterial oxygen saturation <90% and/or pulmonary congestion. Despite lack of proof for long-term benefit of supplementary oxygen, give it to all patients with uncomplicated STEMI as it will benefit patients with unrecognised hypoxia.

Acetylsalicylic acid (ASA)

Large randomised controlled trials indicate decreased mortality when ASA (75–325 mg) is given to hospitalised patients with ACS. A few studies have suggested reduced mortality if ASA is given earlier. Therefore, give ASA as soon as possible to all patients with suspected ACS unless the patient has a known true allergy to ASA. The initial chewed dose of ASA is 160–325 mg. Other forms of ASA (soluble, IV) may be as effective as chewed tablets.

Reperfusion therapy

Reperfusion therapy is the most important advance in the treatment of AMI in the last 20 y. Large clinical trials have proven that fibrinolytic therapy in ACS patients with STEMI or new or presumed new left bundle branch block (LBBB), who present within 12 h of onset of symptoms, reduces short- and long-term mortality. The benefit achieved with fibrinolytic therapy is profoundly time-dependent: it is particularly effective if given within the first 3 h of the onset of symptoms. The efficacy of primary PCI is also time-sensitive but less so than fibrinolysis.

Out-of-hospital fibrinolysis

A meta-analysis of six trials documented a 17% decrease in the mortality among patients treated with out-of-hospital fibrinolysis compared to in-hospital fibrinolysis. The average time gained by out-of-hospital fibrinolysis was 60 min, and the results were independent of the experience of the provider. Thus, giving fibrinolytics out-of-hospital to patients with STEMI or signs and symptoms of an ACS with presumed new LBBB is beneficial. Fibrinolytic therapy can be given safely by trained paramedics, nurses or physicians using an established protocol. The efficacy is greatest within the first 3 h of the onset of symptoms. An effective and safe system for out-of-hospital thrombolytic therapy requires adequate facilities for the diagnosis and treatment of STEMI and its complications. Ideally, there should be a capability of communicating with experienced hospital doctors.

Patients with symptoms of ACS and ECG evidence of STEMI (or presumably new LBBB or true posterior infarction) presenting directly to the emergency department should be given fibrinolytic therapy as soon as possible unless there is immediate access to primary PCI within 90 min.

Risks of fibrinolytic therapy

Healthcare professionals who give fibrinolytic therapy must be aware of its contraindications (Table 4.1) and risks. Patients with large AMIs (e.g. indicated by extensive ECG changes) are likely to derive the greatest benefit from fibrinolytic therapy. Benefits of fibrinolytic therapy are less impressive in inferior wall infarctions than in anterior infarctions. Older patients have an absolute higher risk of death, but the absolute benefit of fibrinolytic therapy is similar to that of younger patients. Patients over 75 y have an increased risk of intracranial bleeding from fibrinolysis; thus, the absolute benefit of thrombolysis is reduced by this complication. The risk of intracranial bleeding

Table 4.1 Contraindications for thrombolysis*

Absolute contraindications
• Haemorrhagic stroke or stroke of unknown origin at any time • Ischaemic stroke in the preceding 6 months • Central nervous system damage or neoplasms • Recent major trauma/surgery/head injury (within the preceding 3 weeks) • Gastrointestinal bleeding within the last month • Known bleeding disorder • Aortic dissection
Relative contraindications
• Transient ischaemic attack in preceding 6 months • Oral anticoagulant therapy • Pregnancy within 1 week post-partum • Non-compressible punctures • Traumatic resuscitation • Refractory hypertension (systolic blood pressure >180 mmHg) • Advanced liver disease • Infective endocarditis • Active peptic ulcer

*According to the guidelines of the European Society of Cardiology.

is increased in patients with a systolic blood pressure of over 180 mmHg; this degree of hypertension is a relative contraindication to fibrinolytic therapy. The intracranial bleeding risk also depends in part on which fibrinolytic drug is used: the total mortality is lower with the more fibrin-specific thrombolytics (alteplase, tenecteplase, reteplase), but the intracranial bleeding risk is lower with streptokinase. The risk of intracranial bleeding is also increased by the use of antithrombotic therapy, particularly heparin.

Primary percutaneous intervention

Coronary angioplasty, with or without stent placement, has become the first-line treatment for patients with STEMI because it has been shown to be superior to fibrinolysis in the combined endpoints of death, stroke and reinfarction in several studies and meta-analyses. This improvement was found when primary PCI was undertaken by a skilled person in a high volume centre (i.e. >75 procedures per operator per year) with a delay of balloon inflation of not more than 90 min after first contact. In the randomised studies comparing primary PCI and fibrinolytic therapy, the typical delay from decision to the beginning of treatment with either primary PCI or fibrinolytic therapy was less than 60 min; however, in registries that reflect standard practice more realistically, the delay was often longer. Two reports comparing fibrinolytic therapy with primary PCI showed no difference in survival if fibrinolytic therapy was initiated within 2 or 3 h of onset of symptoms.

All patients presenting with STEMI and symptoms of ACS and presumably new LBBB presenting within 12 h after onset of symptoms should be evaluated for reperfusion therapy (fibrinolytic therapy or PCI). Primary PCI is preferred in patients with symptom duration of over 3 h, if a skilled team can undertake it within 90 min after first patient contact, and in all patients who have contraindications to fibrinolytic therapy. If the duration of symptoms is less than 3 h, treatment is more time-sensitive and the superiority of out-of-hospital fibrinolytic therapy, immediate in-hospital fibrinolytic therapy or transfer for primary PCI is not yet established clearly.

Triage and interfacility transfer for primary PCI

The risk of death, reinfarction or stroke is reduced if patients with STEMI are transferred promptly from community hospitals to tertiary care facilities for primary PCI. It is unclear whether immediate fibrinolytic therapy (in- or out-of-hospital) or transfer for primary PCI is superior for patients presenting with STEMI with a symptom duration of <2–3 h. Transfer of STEMI patients for primary PCI is reasonable for those presenting later than 3 h but less than 12 h after onset of symptoms, provided that the transfer can be achieved rapidly. Optimally, primary PCI should occur within 90 min from the first contact with the healthcare provider deciding to treat or transfer.

Interfacility transfer for early PCI after fibrinolytic therapy

Older studies, that did not include modern adjunctive drugs and PCI techniques with stenting, do not support a strategy of fibrinolytic therapy combined with early PCI. In contrast, several recent smaller studies support a strategy of in-hospital fibrinolytic therapy in a peripheral hospital followed by transfer for PCI within 24 h of fibrinolytic therapy. The timing of PCI after fibrinolytic therapy, the use of coronary stents and control group interventions differ widely among these trials.

There is insufficient evidence to recommend routine transfer of patients for early PCI after successful fibrinolytic therapy. Transfer for early PCI is recommended for patients in cardiogenic shock, especially for those younger than 75 y, and for those who are haemodynamically unstable or have persistent ischaemic symptoms after fibrinolytic therapy.

Cardiogenic shock

Cardiogenic shock (and to some extent severe left ventricular failure) is one of the complications of ACS and has a mortality rate of more than 50%. Cardiogenic shock in STEMI is not a contraindication to fibrinolytic therapy, but PCI is preferable. Early revascularisation (i.e. primary or facilitated PCI or surgery) is indicated for those patients who develop shock within 36 h after symptom onset of AMI and are suitable for revascularisation.

Suspect right ventricular infarction in patients with inferior infarction, clinical shock and clear lung fields. ST segment elevation ≥1 mm in lead V4R is a useful indicator of right ventricular infarction. These patients have an in-hospital mortality of up to 30% and many benefit greatly from reperfusion therapy (fibrinolytic therapy and/or PCI). Avoid nitrates and other vasodilators, and treat hypotension with intravenous fluid.

Adjunctive treatment in reperfusion therapy in ACS

Heparin

Heparin is an indirect inhibitor of thrombin, which in combination with ASA is used as an adjunct with fibrinolytic therapy or primary PCI and as an important part of treatment of unstable angina and STEMI. Limitations of unfractionated heparin include its unpredictable anticoagulant effect in individual patients, the need for it to be given intravenously and the need to monitor aPTT. Moreover, heparin can induce thrombocytopenia. Low molecular weight heparin has a more predictable anticoagulant effect with lower rates of thrombocytopenia. It can be given subcutaneously in a weight-adjusted dose and does not require laboratory monitoring. Low molecular weight heparins may accumulate in patients with impaired renal function.

Unfractionated heparin (UFH) versus low molecular weight heparin (LMWH) in NSTEMI

In comparison with UFH, LMWH (enoxaparin) reduces the combined endpoint of mortality, myocardial infarction and the need for urgent revascularisation, if given within the first 24–36 h of onset of symptoms of NSTEMI/UAP. Although LMWH increases the incidence of minor bleeding, in comparison with UFH, the incidence of serious bleeding is not increased. Early treatment with LMWH (enoxaparin) is the preferred therapy for patients with NSTEMI/UAP in addition to ASA, whenever a non-interventional strategy is planned. Consider UFH if reperfusion is planned in the first 24–36 h after symptom onset. Optimal target value of aPPT is 50–70 s. Avoid switching between UFH and LMWH because it may increase bleeding complications.

UFH versus LMWH in STEMI

Two large randomised controlled thrombolysis studies comparing LMWH to UFH demonstrated a reduced frequency of ischaemic complications when given to patients with STEMI within 6 h of the onset of symptoms. This must be balanced against the increase in intracranial haemorrhage in patients over 75 y of age receiving LMWH. There is no evidence to support giving LMWH to patients with STEMI proceeding to an invasive strategy. Thus, LMWH is an acceptable alternative to UFH as an ancillary therapy for patients younger than 75 y without significant renal dysfunction who are treated with fibrinolytic therapy. In elderly patients, UFH is recommended as an ancillary therapy to fibrinolytic therapy and for any STEMI patient for whom revascularisation is planned. The optimal target value of aPPT is 50–70 s. The use of heparin (preferably UFH) depends partly on which fibrinolytic drug is used. Heparin is needed after shorter acting drugs because of the rebound hyper-coagulable state that occurs after a few hours, but not with streptokinase because the fibrinolytic effect lasts for about 48 h.

Glycoprotein (Gp) IIb/IIIa inhibitors

The platelet Gp IIb/IIIa receptor is the final common pathway to platelet aggregation. The synthetic substances eptifibatide and tirofiban modulate this receptor activity reversibly, whereas the receptor antibody abciximab blocks it irreversibly.

Gp IIb/IIIa inhibitors in NSTEMI/unstable angina

The incidence of death and recurrent ischaemia is reduced when Gp IIb/IIIa inhibitors are added to standard therapy including ASA and heparin in high-risk patients with UAP/NSTEMI treated with mechanical reperfusion. High-risk features include persistent pain, haemodynamic or rhythm instability, diabetes, acute or dynamic ECG changes and any elevation in cardiac troponins. Tirofiban or eptifibatide failed to reduce death or recurrent ischaemia in patients with UA/NSTEMI without mechanical perfusion but showed a reduction in 30-d mortality in a later meta-analysis. In patients with UA/NSTEMI, abciximab given in addition to standard therapy without mechanical intervention resulted in a trend toward a worse outcome. Therefore, in high-risk patients, give Gp IIb/IIIa inhibitors in addition to standard therapy in patients in whom revascularisation therapy is planned. If revascularisation therapy is not planned, tirofiban and eptifibatide can be given to high-risk NSTEMI/UAP patients in conjunction with ASA and LMWH. Do not give abciximab if PCI is not planned.

Gp IIb/IIIa inhibitors in STEMI

Gp IIb/IIIa receptor blockers in combination with a reduced dose of fibrinolytics do not reduce mortality in patients with STEMI, but increase bleeding risk in patients over 75 y. Abciximab reduces mortality when given to patients with STEMI and planned primary PCI, but is not beneficial in patients not proceeding to primary PCI. Pre-hospital use of abciximab may improve the patency of the infarct-related artery with PCI. There is no benefit in giving tirofiban in addition to standard therapy out of hospital or in the emergency department. Abciximab may be helpful in reducing short-term mortality and short-term reinfarction in patients treated with PCI without fibrinolytic therapy. Abciximab is not recommended in combination with fibrinolytics in patients with STEMI.

Clopidogrel

Clopidogrel inhibits the platelet ADP receptor irreversibly, which further reduces platelet aggregation in addition to that produced by ASA. Compared to ASA, there is no increased risk of bleeding with clopidogrel. If given in addition to heparin and ASA within 4 h of presentation, clopidogrel improves outcome in patients with high-risk ACS. There is a significant reduction in adverse ischaemic events at 28 d after elective PCI when clopidogrel is given at least 6 h before intervention. A recent trial documented a significant reduction in the composite endpoint of an occluded infarct-related artery (TIMI flow grade 0 or 1) on angiography or death or recurrent myocardial infarction before angiography when clopidogrel (300 mg loading dose, followed by 75 mg daily dose up to 8 d in hospital) is given to patients up to 75 y with STEMI who are treated with fibrinolytic therapy, acetylsalicylic acid and heparin.

Give a 300 mg oral loading dose of clopidogrel early, as well as standard care, to patients with ACS if they have an increase in serum cardiac biomarkers and/or new ECG changes consistent with ischaemia when a medical approach or PCI is planned. Give clopidogrel to patients with STEMI up to 75 y receiving fibrinolytic therapy, ASA and heparin.

Clopidogrel 300 mg can be given instead of ASA to patients with a suspected ACS who have a true allergy to or gastrointestinal intolerance of ASA.

Primary and secondary prevention interventions

Beta-blockers

Several studies, undertaken mainly in the pre-reperfusion era, indicate a decreased mortality, incidence of reinfarction and cardiac rupture as well as a lower incidence of ventricular fibrillation and supraventricular arrhythmia in patients treated early with a beta-blocker. Intravenous beta-blockade may also reduce mortality in patients undergoing primary PCI who are not on oral beta-blockers.

Haemodynamically stable patients presenting with an ACS should be given intravenous beta-blockers promptly, followed by regular oral therapy unless contraindicated or poorly tolerated. Contraindications to beta-blockers include hypotension, bradycardia, second or third degree AV block, moderate to severe congestive heart failure and severe reactive airway disease. Give a beta-blocker irrespective of the need for early revascularisation therapy.

Anti-arrhythmics

Apart from the use of a beta-blocker, there is no evidence to support the use of anti-arrhythmic prophylaxis after ACS. Ventricular fibrillation (VF) accounts for most of the early deaths from ACS; the incidence of VF is highest in the first hour after onset of symptoms. This explains why numerous studies have been performed with the aim of demonstrating the prophylactic effect of anti-arrhythmic therapy. The effects of anti-arrhythmic drugs (lidocaine, magnesium, disopyramide, mexiletine, verapamil) given prophylactically to patients with ACS have been studied. Prophylaxis with lidocaine reduces the incidence of VF but may increase mortality. Routine treatment with magnesium in patients with AMI does not improve mortality. Arrhythmia prophylaxis using disopyramide, mexiletine or verapamil, given within the first hours of an ACS, does not improve mortality. In contrast, intravenous beta-blockers reduced the incidence of VF when given to patients with ACS.

Angiotensin-converting enzyme inhibitors and angiotensin-II receptor blockers

Oral ACE inhibitors reduce mortality when given to patients with acute myocardial infarction with or without early reperfusion therapy. The beneficial effects are most pronounced in patients presenting with anterior infarction, pulmonary congestion or left ventricular ejection fraction <40%. Do not give ACE inhibitors if the systolic blood pressure is less than 100 mmHg at admission or if there is a known contraindication to these drugs. A trend towards higher mortality has been documented if an intravenous ACE inhibitor is started within the first 24 h after onset of symptoms.

Therefore, give an oral ACE inhibitor within 24 h after symptom onset in patients with AMI regardless of whether early reperfusion therapy is planned, particularly in those patients with anterior infarction, pulmonary congestion or left ventricular ejection fraction below 40%. Do not give intravenous ACE inhibitors within 24 h of onset of symptoms. Give an angiotensin receptor blocker (ARB) to patients intolerant of ACE inhibitors.

Statins

Statins reduce the incidence of major adverse cardiovascular events when given within a few days after onset of ACS. Start statin therapy within 24 h of onset of symptoms of ACS. If patients are already on statin therapy, do not stop it.

Further reading

1. International Liaison Committee on Resuscitation. 2005 International Consensus on Cardiopulmonary Resuscitation and Emergency Cardiovascular Care Science with Treatment Recommendations. Resuscitation 2005;67:249–69.
2. European Resuscitation Council. European Resuscitation Council guidelines for resuscitation 2005. Resuscitation 2005;67(Suppl 1):S87–96.

Chapter 5
Paediatric life support

Dominique Biarent, Robert Bingham, Sam Richmond, Ian Maconachie, Jonathan Wyllie, Shelia Simpson, Antonio Rodriguez Nunez and David Zideman

Paediatric basic life support

Guidelines changes

The current revision has a strong focus on simplification, based on the knowledge that many children receive no resuscitation at all because rescuers fear doing harm. This fear is fuelled by the knowledge that resuscitation guidelines for children are different. Consequently, a major area of study was the feasibility of applying the same guidance for all adults and children. Bystander resuscitation improves outcome significantly and there is good evidence from paediatric animal models that even doing chest compressions or expired air ventilation alone may result in better outcome than doing nothing at all. It follows that outcomes could be improved if bystanders who would otherwise do nothing were encouraged to begin resuscitation, even if they are not following an algorithm targeted specifically at children. There are, however, distinct differences between the predominantly adult arrest of cardiac origin and asphyxial arrest, which is most common in children, so a separate paediatric algorithm is justified for those with a duty to respond to paediatric emergencies (usually health professionals), who are also in a position to receive enhanced training.

Compression:ventilation ratios

The ILCOR treatment recommendation was that the compression:ventilation ratio should be based on whether one or more rescuers were present. ILCOR recommends that lay rescuers, who usually learn only single rescuer techniques, should be taught to use a ratio of 30 compressions to two ventilations, which is the same as the adult guidelines and enables anyone trained in BLS techniques to resuscitate children with minimal additional information. Two or more rescuers with a duty to respond should learn a different ratio (15:2) as this has been validated by animal and manikin studies. This latter group, who would normally be health professionals, should be in a position to receive enhanced training targeted specifically at the resuscitation of children. Although there are no data to support the superiority of any particular ratio in children, ratios of between 5:1 and 15:2 have been studied in manikins, and animal and mathematical models, and there is increasing evidence that the 5:1 ratio delivers an inadequate number of compressions. There is certainly no justification for having two separate ratios for children greater or less than 8 y, so a single ratio of 15:2 for multiple rescuers with a duty to respond is a logical simplification.

It would certainly negate any benefit of simplicity if lay rescuers were taught a different ratio for use if there were two of them, but those with a duty to respond can use the 30:2 ratio if they are alone, particularly if they are not achieving an adequate number of compressions because of difficulty in the transition between ventilation and compression.

Age definitions

The adoption of single compression:ventilation ratios for children of all ages, together with the change in advice on the lower age limit for the use of automated external defibrillators (AEDs), renders the previous guideline division between children above and below 8 y unnecessary. The onset of puberty, which is the physiological end of childhood, is the most logical landmark for the upper age limit for use of paediatric guidance. Clearly, it is inappropriate and unnecessary to establish the onset of puberty formally; if the rescuer believes the victim to be a child then they should use the paediatric guidelines.

It is necessary to differentiate between infants (less than 1 y) and older children, as there are some important differences between these two groups.

Chest compression technique

The modification to age definitions enables a simplification of the advice on chest compression. Advice for determining the landmarks for infant compression is now the same as for older children, as there is evidence that the previous recommendation could result in compression over the upper abdomen. Infant compression technique remains the same: two-finger compression for single rescuers and two-thumb, encircling technique for two or more rescuers, but for older children there is no division between one- or two-hand techniques. The emphasis is on achieving an adequate depth of compression with minimal interruptions using one or two hands according to rescuer preference.

Foreign body airway obstruction sequence

The guidance for managing foreign body airway obstruction (FBAO) in children has been simplified and brought into closer alignment to the adult sequence.

Definitions

An **infant** is a child under 1 y. A **child** is between 1 y and puberty. It is neither appropriate nor necessary to establish the onset of puberty formally. If the rescuer believes the victim to be a child then they should use the paediatric guidelines.

Sequence of action

Rescuers who have been taught adult BLS and have no specific knowledge of paediatric resuscitation may use the adult sequence with the exception that they should perform five initial breaths followed by approximately 1 min of CPR before they go for help (see adult BLS guidelines) (Figure 5.1).

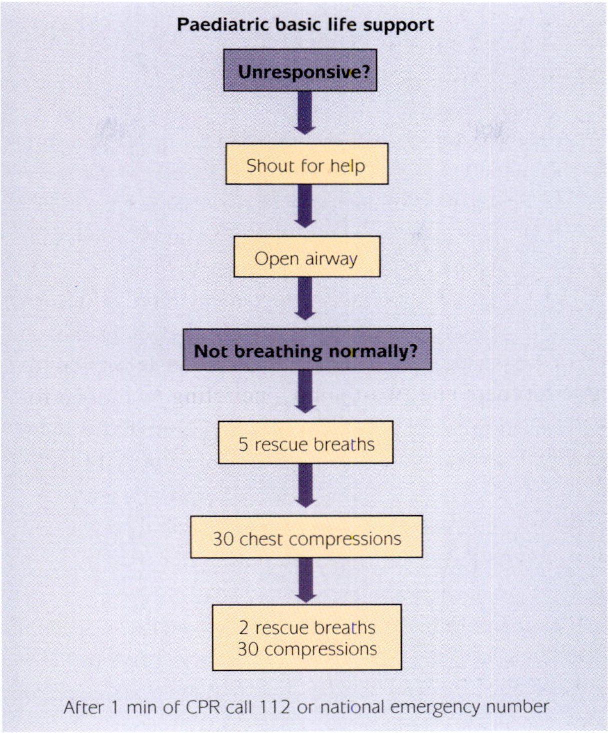

Figure 5.1. Paediatric basic life support algorithm.

The following sequence is to be followed by those with a duty to respond to paediatric emergencies (usually health professionals):

1. **Ensure the safety of rescuer and child.**
2. **Check the child's responsiveness.**

- Gently stimulate the child and ask loudly: "Are you all right?"
- Do not shake infants and children with suspected cervical spinal injuries.

3A. If the child responds by answering or moving:

- Leave the child in the position in which you find him (provided he is not in further danger).

- Check his condition and get help if needed.
- Reassess him regularly.

3B. If the child does not respond:

- Shout for help.
- Open the child's airway by tilting the head and lifting the chin.
    - Initially with the child in the position in which you find him, place your hand on his forehead and gently tilt his head back.
    - At the same time, with your fingertip(s) under the point of the child's chin, lift the chin. Do not push on the soft tissues under the chin as this may block the airway.
    - If you still have difficulty in opening the airway, try the jaw thrust method: place the first two fingers of each hand behind each side of the child's mandible and push the jaw forward.
    - Both methods may be easier if the child is turned carefully onto his back.

If you suspect that there may have been an injury to the neck, try to open the airway using chin lift or jaw thrust alone. If this is unsuccessful, add head tilt a small amount at a time until the airway is open.

4. Keeping the airway open, look, listen and feel for normal breathing by putting your face close to the child's face and looking along the chest:

- **Look** for chest movements.
- **Listen** at the child's nose and mouth for breath sounds.
- **Feel** for air movement on your cheek.

Look, listen and feel for no more than 10 s before deciding:

5A. If the child is breathing normally:

- Turn the child on his side into the recovery position (see below).
- Check for continued breathing.

5B. If the child is *not* breathing or is making agonal gasps (infrequent, irregular breaths):

- Carefully remove any obvious airway obstruction.

- Give five initial rescue breaths.
- While performing the rescue breaths note any gag or cough response to your action. These responses or their absence will form part of your assessment of 'signs of a circulation', which will be described later.

Rescue breaths for a child over 1 y of age (Figure 5.2):

- Ensure head tilt and chin lift.
- Pinch the soft part of the nose closed with the index finger and thumb of your hand on his forehead.
- Open his mouth a little, but maintain the chin upwards.
- Take a breath and place your lips around the mouth, making sure that you have a good seal.
- Blow steadily into the mouth over about 1–1.5 s watching for chest rise.
- Maintain head tilt and chin lift, take your mouth away from the victim and watch for his chest to fall as air comes out.
- Take another breath and repeat this sequence five times. Identify effectiveness by seeing that the child's chest has risen and fallen in a similar fashion to the movement produced by a normal breath.

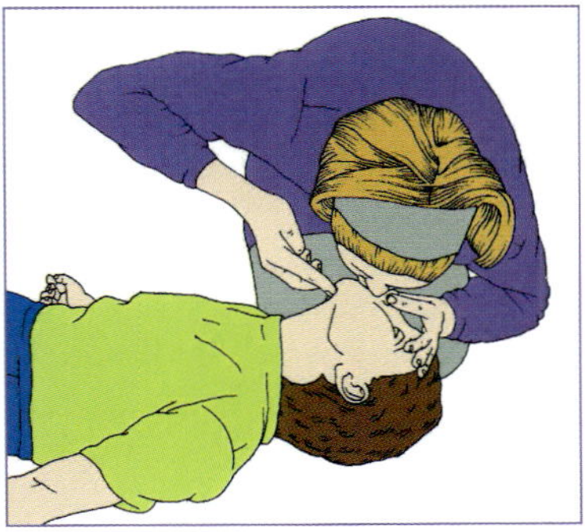

Figure 5.2. Mouth-to-mouth ventilation – child. © ERC 2005.

Rescue breaths for an infant (Figure 5.3):

- Ensure a neutral position of the head and a chin lift.
- Take a breath and cover the mouth and nasal apertures of the infant with your mouth, making sure you have a good seal. If the nose and mouth cannot be covered in

the older infant, the rescuer may attempt to seal only the infant's nose or mouth with his mouth (if the nose is used, close the lips to prevent air escape).

- Blow steadily into the infant's mouth and nose over 1–1.5 s, sufficient to make the chest visibly rise.
- Maintain head tilt and chin lift, take your mouth away from the victim and watch for his chest to fall as air comes out.
- Take another breath and repeat this sequence five times. If you have difficulty achieving an effective breath, the airway may be obstructed:
- Open the child's mouth and remove any visible obstruction. Do not perform a blind finger sweep.
- Ensure that there is adequate head tilt and chin lift but also that the neck is not over extended.
- If head tilt and chin lift has not opened the airway, try the jaw thrust method.
- Make up to five attempts to achieve effective breaths. If still unsuccessful, move on to chest compressions.

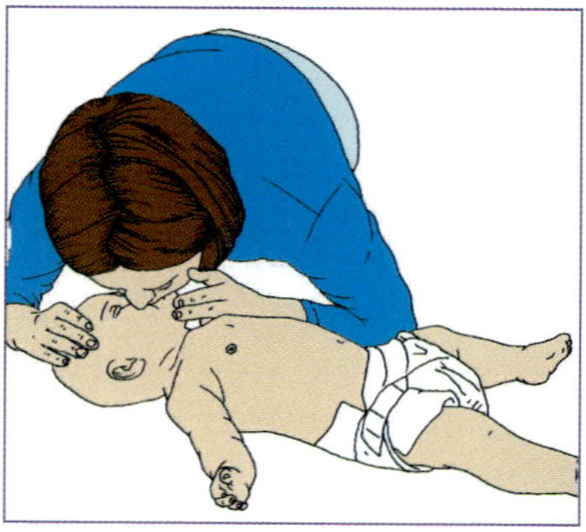

Figure 5.3. Mouth-to-mouth and nose ventilation – infant. © ERC 2005..

6. Assess the child's circulation. Take no more than 10 s to:

- Look for signs of a circulation. This includes any movement, coughing or normal breathing (not agonal gasps – these are infrequent, irregular breaths).
- Check the pulse (if you are a healthcare provider) but ensure you take no more than 10 s.

- **In a child over 1 year** – feel for the carotid pulse in the neck.
- **In an infant** – feel for the brachial pulse on the inner aspect of the upper arm.

7A. If you are confident that you can detect signs of a circulation within 10 s:

- Continue rescue breathing, if necessary, until the child starts breathing effectively on his own.
- Turn the child on to his side (into the recovery position) if he remains unconscious.
- Reassess the child frequently.

7B. If there are no signs of a circulation, or no pulse or a slow pulse (less than 60 min^{-1} with poor perfusion), or you are not sure:

- Start chest compressions.
- Combine rescue breathing and chest compressions:
    - **Chest compressions**
      For all children, compress the lower third of the sternum. To avoid compressing the upper abdomen, locate the xiphisternum by finding the angle where the lowest ribs join in the middle. Compress the sternum one finger's breadth above this; the compression should be sufficient to depress it by approximately one-third of the depth of the chest. Release the pressure and repeat at a rate of about 100 min^{-1}. After 15 compressions, tilt the head, lift the chin and give two effective breaths. Continue compressions and breaths in a ratio of 15:2. Lone rescuers may use a ratio of 30:2, particularly if having difficulty with the transition between compression and ventilation. Although the rate of compressions will be 100 times per minute, the actual number delivered per minute will be less than 100 because of pauses to give breaths. The best method for compression varies slightly between infants and children.
    - **Chest compression in infants** (Figure 5.4)
      The lone rescuer compresses the sternum with

the tips of two fingers. If there are two or more rescuers, use the encircling technique. Place both thumbs flat side by side on the lower third of the sternum (as above) with the tips pointing towards the infant's head. Spread the rest of both hands with the fingers together to encircle the lower part of the infant's rib cage with the tips of the fingers supporting the infant's back. Press down on the lower sternum with the two thumbs to depress it approximately one-third of the depth of the infant's chest.

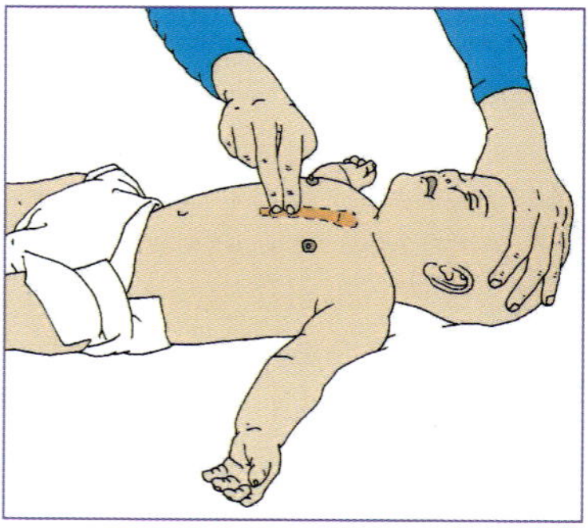

Figure 5.4. Chest compression – infant. © ERC 2005.

- **Chest compression in children over 1 y of age** (Figures 5.5 and 5.6)
  Place the heel of one hand over the lower third of the sternum (as above). Lift the fingers to ensure that pressure is not applied over the child's ribs. Position yourself vertically above the victim's chest and, with your arm straight, compress the sternum to depress it by approximately one-third of the depth of the chest. In larger children or for small rescuers, this is achieved most easily by using both hands with the fingers interlocked.

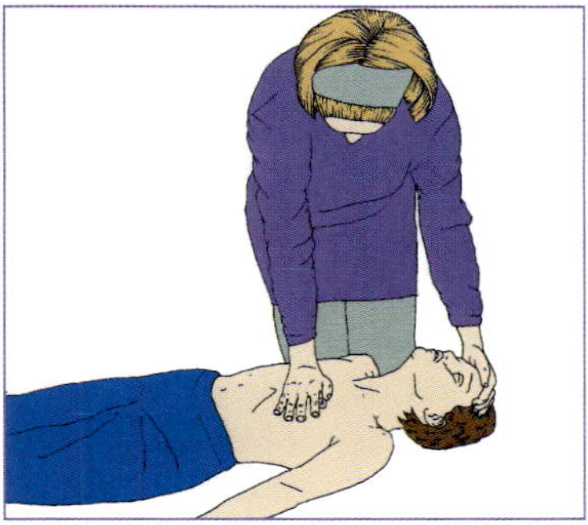

Figure 5.5. Chest compression, one hand – child. © ERC 2005.

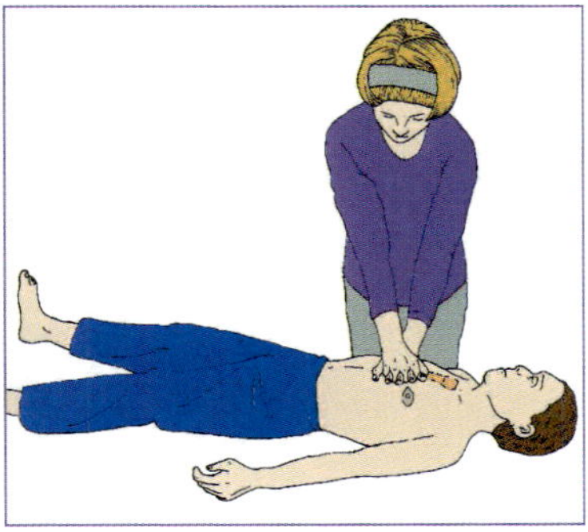

Figure 5.6. Chest compression, two hands – child. © ERC 2005.

8. Continue resuscitation until:

- The child shows signs of life (spontaneous respiration, pulse, movement).
- Qualified help arrives.
- You become exhausted.

When to call for assistance

It is vital for rescuers to get help as quickly as possible when a child collapses:

- When more than one rescuer is available, one starts resuscitation while another rescuer goes for assistance.

- If only one rescuer is present, undertake resuscitation for about *1 min* before going for assistance. To minimise interruption in CPR, it may be possible to carry an infant or small child whilst summoning help.
- The only exception to performing 1 min of CPR before going for help is in the case of a child with a *witnessed, sudden* collapse when the rescuer is alone. In this case cardiac arrest is likely to be arrhythmogenic in origin and the child will need defibrillation. Seek help immediately *if there is no-one to go for you.*

Recovery position

An unconscious child whose airway is clear, and who is breathing spontaneously, should be turned on his side into the recovery position. There are several recovery positions; each has its advocates. The important principles to be followed are:

- Place the child in as near true lateral position as possible with his mouth dependent to enable free drainage of fluid.
- The position should be stable. In an infant this may require the support of a small pillow or a rolled up blanket placed behind the back to maintain the position.
- Avoid any pressure on the chest that impairs breathing.
- It should be possible to turn the child on to his side and to return him back easily and safely, taking into consideration the possibility of cervical spine injury.
- Ensure the airway can be observed and accessed easily.
- The adult recovery position is suitable for use in children.

Foreign body airway obstruction (FBAO)

No new evidence on this subject was presented during the 2005 Consensus Conference. Back blows, chest thrusts and abdominal thrusts all increase intrathoracic pressure and can expel foreign bodies from the airway. In half of the episodes more than one technique is needed to relieve the obstruction.

There are no data to indicate which measure should be used first or in which order they should be applied. If one is unsuccessful, try the others in rotation until the object is cleared.

The International Guidelines 2000 algorithm is difficult to teach and knowledge retention poor. The FBAO algorithm for children has been simplified and aligned with the adult version. This should improve skill retention and encourage people, who might otherwise have been reluctant, to perform FBAO manoeuvres on children.

The most significant difference from the adult algorithm is that abdominal thrusts should not be used to treat choking infants. Although abdominal thrusts have caused injuries in all age groups, the risk is particularly high in infants and very young children. This is because of the horizontal position of the ribs, which leaves the upper abdominal viscera much more exposed to trauma. For this reason, the guidelines for the treatment of FBAO are different between infants and children.

Recognition of FBAO

When a foreign body enters the airway the child reacts immediately by coughing in an attempt to expel it. A spontaneous cough is likely to be more effective and safer than any manoeuvre a rescuer might perform. However, if coughing is absent or ineffective and the object completely obstructs the airway, the child will rapidly become asphyxiated. Active interventions to relieve FBAO are therefore required only when coughing becomes ineffective, but they then need to be commenced rapidly and confidently.

The majority of choking events in infants and children occur during play or eating episodes when a carer is usually present; thus, the events are frequently witnessed and interventions are usually initiated when the child is conscious.

Foreign body airway obstruction is characterised by the sudden onset of respiratory distress associated with coughing, gagging or stridor. Similar signs and symptoms may be associated with other causes of airway obstruction such as laryngitis or epiglottitis, which require different management.

Suspect FBAO if the onset was very sudden and there are no other signs of illness and if there are clues to alert the rescuer, e.g. a history of eating or playing with small items immediately before the onset of symptoms (see Table 5.1).

Table 5.1 Differentiation between ineffective and effective coughing in FBAO

General signs of FBAO	
• Witnessed episode • Coughing/choking • Sudden onset • Recent history of playing with/eating small objects	
Ineffective coughing	**Effective coughing**
• Unable to vocalise • Quiet or silent cough • Unable to breathe • Cyanosis • Decreasing level of consciousness	• Crying or verbal response to questions • Loud cough • Able to take a breath before coughing • Fully responsive

Relief of FBAO

1. Safety and summoning assistance

Safety is paramount: rescuers must not place themselves in danger and should consider the safest treatment of the choking child.

- If the child is coughing effectively, no external manoeuvre is necessary. Encourage the child to cough, and monitor continually.
- If the child's coughing is (or is becoming) ineffective, *shout for help* immediately and determine the child's conscious level.

2. Conscious child with FBAO

- If the child is still conscious but has absent or ineffective coughing, give back blows.
- If back blows do not relieve the FBAO, give chest thrusts to infants or abdominal thrusts to children. These manoeuvres create an 'artificial cough' to increase intrathoracic pressure and dislodge the foreign body.

Back blows

- **The infant**
  - Support the infant in a head downwards, prone position, to enable gravity to assist removal of the foreign body.
  - A seated or kneeling rescuer should be able to support the infant safely across their lap.
  - Support the infant's head by placing the thumb of one hand, at the angle of the lower jaw, and one or two fingers from the same hand, at the same point on the other side of the jaw.
  - Do not compress the soft tissues under the infant's jaw, as this will exacerbate the airway obstruction.
  - Deliver up to five sharp back blows with the heel of one hand in the middle of the back between the shoulder blades.
  - The aim is too relieve the obstruction with each blow rather than to give all five.
- **The child over 1 year**
  - Back blows are more effective if the child is positioned head down.
  - A small child may be placed across the rescuer's lap as with the infant.
  - If this is not possible, support the child in a forward leaning position and deliver the back blows from behind.

If back blows fail to dislodge the object, and the child is still conscious, use chest thrusts for infants or abdominal thrusts for children. *Do not use abdominal thrusts (Heimlich manoeuvre) in infants.*

Chest thrusts for infants

- Turn the infant into a head downwards supine position. This is achieved safely by placing the free arm along the infant's back and encircling the occiput with the hand.
- Support the infant down your arm, which is placed down (or across) your thigh.

- Identify the landmark for chest compressions (lower sternum approximately a finger's breadth above the xiphisternum).
- Give five chest thrusts; these are similar to chest compressions but sharper and delivered at a slower rate.

Abdominal thrusts for children over 1 y

- Stand or kneel behind the child; place your arms under the child's arms and encircle his torso.
- Clench your fist and place it between the umbilicus and xiphisternum.
- Grasp this hand with the other hand and pull sharply inwards and upwards.
- Repeat up to five times.
- Ensure that pressure is not applied to the xiphoid process or the lower rib cage – this may cause abdominal trauma.

Following the chest or abdominal thrusts, reassess the child. If the object has not been expelled and the victim is still conscious, continue the sequence of back blows and chest (for infant) or abdominal (for children) thrusts. Call out, or send, for help if it is still not available. Do not leave the child at this stage.

If the object is expelled successfully, assess the child's clinical condition. It is possible that part of the object may remain in the respiratory tract and cause complications. If there is any doubt, seek medical assistance. Abdominal thrusts may cause internal injuries and all victims so treated should be examined by a medical practitioner.

3. Unconscious child with FBAO

If the child with FBAO is, or becomes, unconscious, place him on a firm, flat surface. Call out, or send, for help if it is still not available. Do not leave the child at this stage, proceed as follows:

Airway opening

Open the mouth and look for any obvious object. If one is seen, make an attempt to remove it with a single finger sweep.

Do not attempt blind or repeated finger sweeps – these can impact the object more deeply into the pharynx and cause injury.

Rescue breaths

Open the airway using a head tilt/chin lift and attempt five rescue breaths. Assess the effectiveness of each breath: if a breath does not make the chest rise, reposition the head before making the next attempt.

Chest compressions and CPR (see Figure 5.7)

- Attempt five rescue breaths and if there is no response (moving, coughing, spontaneous breaths) proceed to chest compressions without further assessment of the circulation.
- Follow the sequence for single rescuer CPR (step 7B above) for approximately a minute before summoning the EMS (if this has not already been done by someone else).
- When the airway is opened for attempted delivery of rescue breaths, look to see if the foreign body can be seen in the mouth.
- If an object is seen, attempt to remove it with a single finger sweep.
- If it appears the obstruction has been relieved, open and check the airway as above; deliver rescue breaths if the child is not breathing.
- If the child regains consciousness and exhibits spontaneous effective breathing, place him in a safe side-lying (recovery) position and monitor breathing and conscious level whilst awaiting the arrival of the EMS.

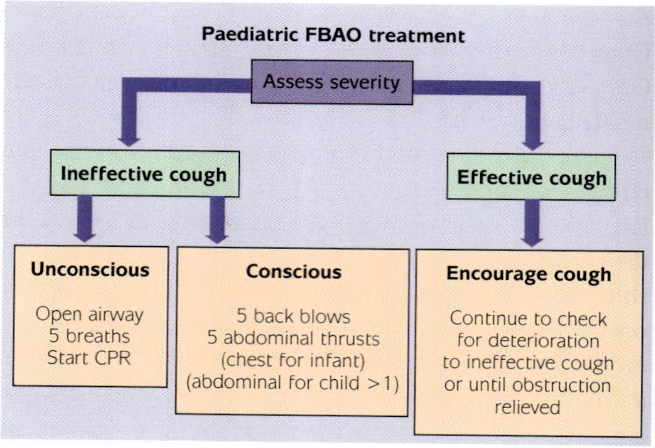

Figure 5.7. Foreign body airway obstruction algorithm.

Paediatric advanced life support

Management of respiratory and circulatory failure

A and B **Open the airway and ensure adequate ventilation and oxygenation.**

- Deliver high flow oxygen.
- Achieving adequate ventilation and oxygenation may include the use of airway adjuncts, bag-mask ventilation (BMV), use of a laryngeal mask airway (LMA), securing a definitive airway by tracheal intubation and positive pressure ventilation.
- In rare, extreme circumstances, a surgical airway may be required.

C **Establish cardiac monitoring.**

- Secure vascular access to the circulation. This may be via peripheral or central intravenous (IV) or by intraosseous (IO) cannulation.
- Give a fluid bolus and/or inotropes as required.

(Re)Assess the child continuously, each time commencing at **A**irway before **B**reathing, thereafter moving onto the **C**irculation.

Airway

Open the airway using basic life support techniques. Oropharyngeal and nasopharyngeal airway adjuncts can help maintain the airway.

Use the oropharyngeal airway *only* in the unconscious child, in whom there is no gag reflex. Use the appropriate size to avoid pushing the tongue backward and obstructing the epiglottis, or directly compressing the glottic area. The soft palate in the child can be damaged by insertion of the oropharyngeal airway; avoid this by inserting the oropharyngeal airway under direct vision and passing it over a tongue depressor or laryngoscope. The nasopharyngeal airway is tolerated better in the conscious child (who has an effective gag reflex), but should not be used if there is a basal skull fracture or a coagulopathy.

These simple airway adjuncts do not protect the airway from aspiration of secretions, blood or stomach contents.

Laryngeal mask airway (LMA)

The LMA is an acceptable initial airway device for providers experienced in its use. It may be particularly helpful in airway obstruction caused by upper airway abnormalities. The LMA does not, however, protect the airway from aspiration of secretions, blood or stomach contents, and therefore close observation is required. LMA use is associated with a higher incidence of complications in small children compared with adults.

Tracheal intubation

Tracheal intubation is the most secure and effective way to establish and maintain the airway, prevent gastric distension, protect the lungs against pulmonary aspiration, enable optimal control of the airway pressure and provide positive end expiratory pressure (PEEP).

The oral route is preferable during resuscitation. Oral intubation is usually quicker and is associated with fewer complications than nasal placement. The judicious use of anaesthetics, sedatives and neuromuscular blocking drugs is indicated in the conscious child to avoid multiple intubation attempts or intubation failure. The anatomy of a child's airway differs significantly from that of an adult; hence, intubation of a child requires special training and experience. Check that tracheal tube placement is correct by clinical examination and end tidal capnography. The tracheal tube must be secured and monitoring of the vital signs is essential.

It is essential to plan an alternative airway management technique in case the trachea cannot be intubated.

Rapid sequence induction and intubation

The child who is in cardiopulmonary arrest and deep coma does not require sedation or analgesia to be intubated; otherwise intubation must be preceded by oxygenation, rapid sedation, analgesia and the use of neuromuscular blocking drugs to minimise intubation complications and failure. The intubator must be experienced and familiar with rapid sequence induction drugs.

Tracheal tube sizes

The tracheal tube internal diameters (ID), in millimetres, for different ages are:

- **Neonates**: 2.5 to 3.5 according to the formula (gestational age in weeks/10).
- **Infants**: 4 or 4.5.
- **Children older than 1 y**: the internal diameter (in mm) = [age in years/4 + 4].

Tracheal tube size estimation according to the length of the child's body as measured by resuscitation tapes is more accurate than using the above formulae.

Cuffed versus uncuffed tracheal tubes

In the pre-hospital setting, an uncuffed tracheal tube may be preferable when using sizes of up to 5.5 mm ID (i.e. up to 8 y of age). In hospital, a cuffed tracheal tube may be useful in certain circumstances, e.g. in cases of poor lung compliance, high airway resistance or large glottic air leak.

The correctly sized cuffed tracheal tube is as safe as an uncuffed tube for infants and children (not for neonates) provided attention is paid to its placement, size and cuff inflation pressure: excessive cuff pressure can lead to ischaemic necrosis of the surrounding laryngeal tissue and stenosis. Maintain the cuff inflation pressure below 20 cm H_2O and check it regularly.

Confirmation of correct tracheal tube placement

Displaced, misplaced or obstructed tubes occur frequently in the intubated child and are associated with increased risk of death. No single technique is 100% reliable for distinguishing oesophageal from tracheal intubation.

Assessment of the correct tracheal tube position is made by:

- Observation of the tube passing beyond the vocal cords.
- Observation of symmetrical chest wall movement during positive pressure ventilation.
- Observation of mist in the tube during the expiratory phase of ventilation.
- Absence of gastric distension.
- Equal air entry heard on bilateral auscultation of both axillae and apices of the chest.
- Absence of air entry into the stomach on auscultation.
- Detection of end tidal CO_2 if the child has a perfusing rhythm (this may be seen with effective CPR).
- Improvement or stabilisation of SpO_2 to the expected range.
- Improvement of heart rate towards the age expected value (or remaining within the normal range).

If the child is in cardiopulmonary arrest and exhaled CO_2 is not detected, or if there is any doubt, confirm tracheal tube position by direct laryngoscopy. After correct placement and confirmation, secure the tracheal tube and reassess its position. Maintain the child's head in neutral position. Flexion of the head drives the tube further into the trachea whereas extension may pull it out of the airway. Confirm the position of the tracheal tube at mid-trachea by chest X-ray; the tracheal tube tip should be at the level of the second or third thoracic vertebra.

DOPES is a useful acronym for the causes of sudden deterioration in an intubated child:

- **D**isplacement of the tracheal tube.
- **O**bstruction of the tracheal tube.
- **P**neumothorax.
- **E**quipment failure (source of gas, BMV, ventilator, etc.).
- **S**tomach (gastric distension may alter diaphragm mechanics).

Breathing

Oxygenation

Use oxygen at the highest concentration (i.e. 100%) during resuscitation. Once circulation is restored, give sufficient oxygen to maintain peripheral oxygen saturation at or above 95%.

Studies in neonates suggest some advantages of using room air during resuscitation but the evidence as yet is inconclusive. In the older child, there is no evidence for any such advantages, so use 100% oxygen for resuscitation.

Ventilation

Healthcare providers commonly provide excessive ventilation to victims of cardiopulmonary or respiratory arrest and this may be detrimental. Hyperventilation causes increased thoracic pressure, decreased cerebral and coronary perfusion, and poorer survival rates in animals and adults. The ideal tidal volume should achieve modest chest wall rise. Use a ratio of 15 chest compressions to two ventilations (a lone rescuer may use 30:2); the correct compression rate is 100 min^{-1}.

Once the airway is protected by tracheal intubation, continue positive pressure ventilation at 12–20 breaths min^{-1} without interrupting chest compressions. Take care to ensure that lung inflation is adequate during chest compressions. When circulation is restored, or if the child still has a perfusing rhythm, ventilate at 12–20 breaths min^{-1} to achieve a normal pCO_2. Hyperventilation is harmful.

Bag-mask ventilation (BMV)

Bag-mask ventilation (BMV) is effective and safe for a child requiring assisted ventilation for a short period, i.e. in the pre-hospital setting or in an emergency department. Assess the effectiveness of BMV by observing adequate chest rise, monitoring heart rate and auscultating for breath sounds, and measuring peripheral oxygen saturation (SpO_2).

Any healthcare provider dealing with children must be able to deliver BMV effectively.

Prolonged ventilation

If prolonged ventilation is required, the benefits of a secured airway probably overcome the potential risks associated with tracheal intubation.

Monitoring of breathing and ventilation

End tidal CO_2

Monitoring end tidal CO_2 with a colorimetric detector or capnometer confirms tracheal tube placement in the child weighing more than 2 kg, and may be used in pre- and in-hospital settings, as well as during any transportation of the child. A colour change or the presence of a capnographic waveform indicates that the tube is in the tracheobronchial tree, both in the presence of a perfusing rhythm and during cardiopulmonary arrest. Capnography does not rule out intubation of the right mainstem bronchus. The absence of exhaled CO_2 during cardiopulmonary arrest may not be caused by tube misplacement since a low or absent end tidal CO_2 may reflect low or absent pulmonary blood flow.

Oesophageal detector devices

The self-inflating bulb or aspirating syringe (oesophageal detector device, ODD) may be used for the secondary confirmation of tracheal tube placement in children with a perfusing rhythm. There are no studies on the use of ODD in children who are in cardiopulmonary arrest.

Pulse oximetry

Clinical evaluation of the oxygen level is unreliable; therefore, monitor the child's peripheral oxygen saturation continuously by pulse oximetry. Pulse oximetry can be unreliable under certain conditions, e.g. if the child is in shock, in cardiopulmonary arrest or has poor peripheral perfusion. Although pulse oximetry is relatively simple, it is a poor guide to tracheal tube displacement; capnography detects tracheal tube dislodgement more rapidly than pulse oximetry.

Circulation

Vascular access

Vascular access is essential to give drugs and fluids, and obtain blood samples. Venous access can be difficult to establish during resuscitation of an infant or child. Limit the maximum number of attempts to obtain intravenous (IV) access to three; thereafter, insert an intraosseous (IO) needle.

Intraosseous access

Intraosseous access is a rapid, safe and effective route to give drugs, fluids and blood products. The onset of action and time to achieve adequate plasma drug concentrations are similar to those provided by central venous access. Bone marrow samples can be used to cross match for blood type or group, for chemical analysis and for blood gas measurement (the values are comparable to central venous blood gases). Flush each drug with a bolus of normal saline to ensure dispersal beyond the marrow cavity, and to achieve faster distribution to the central circulation. Inject large boluses of fluid using manual pressure. Intraosseous access can be maintained until definitive IV access has been established.

Intravenous access

Peripheral IV access provides plasma concentrations of drugs and clinical responses equivalent to central or IO access. Central lines provide more secure long-term access but offer no advantages during resuscitation, compared with IO or peripheral IV access.

Tracheal tube access

Intravenous and IO access are better than the tracheal route for giving drugs. Lipid-soluble drugs, such as lidocaine, atropine, adrenaline and naloxone, are absorbed via the lower airway. Optimal tracheal tube drug doses are unknown because of the great variability of alveolar drug absorption, but the following dosages have been recommended as guidance:

- Adrenaline 100 mcg kg^{-1}
- Lidocaine 2–3 mg kg^{-1}
- Atropine 30 mcg kg^{-1}
- The optimal dose of naloxone is not known.

Dilute the drug in 5 ml of normal saline and follow administration with five ventilations. Do not give non-lipid-soluble medications (e.g. glucose, bicarbonate, calcium) via the tracheal tube because they will damage the airway mucosa.

Fluids and drugs

Volume expansion is indicated when a child shows signs of shock in the absence of volume overload. If systemic perfusion is inadequate, give a bolus of 20 ml kg^{-1} of an isotonic crystalloid even if the systemic blood pressure is normal. Following every bolus, reassess the child's clinical state, using ABC, to decide whether a further bolus or other treatment is required.

There are insufficient data to make recommendations about the use of hypertonic saline for shock associated with head injuries or hypovolaemia. There are also insufficient data to recommend delayed fluid resuscitation in the hypotensive child with blunt trauma. Avoid dextrose-containing solutions unless there is hypoglycaemia. Hypoglycaemia must be actively sought and treated, especially in the small child or infant.

Adenosine

Adenosine is recommended for the treatment of supraventricular tachycardia (SVT). It is safe to use as it has a short half-life (10 s); give it intravenously via upper limb or central veins to minimise the time taken to reach the heart. Give adenosine rapidly, followed by a flush of 3–5 ml of normal saline.

Adrenaline (epinephrine)

The recommended IV/IO dose of adrenaline in children is 10 mcg kg^{-1}. The dose of adrenaline given via the tracheal tube is 10 times this (100 mcg kg^{-1}). If needed, give further doses of adrenaline every 3–5 min.

The use of higher doses of adrenaline via the IV or IO route is not recommended routinely as it does not improve survival or neurological outcome after cardiopulmonary arrest.

Once spontaneous circulation is restored, a continuous infusion of adrenaline may be required. Its haemodynamic effects are dose-related; there is also considerable variability between children in response; therefore, titrate the infusion dose to the desired effect.

To avoid tissue damage it is essential to give adrenaline through a secure intravascular line (IV or IO). Adrenaline (and other catecholamines) is inactivated by alkaline solutions and should never be mixed with sodium bicarbonate.

Amiodarone

Amiodarone is a non-competitive inhibitor of adrenergic receptors. Amiodarone must be injected slowly (over 10–20 min) with systemic blood pressure and ECG monitoring to avoid fast infusion-related hypotension, except when given for the treatment of refractory ventricular fibrillation (VF)/pulseless ventricular tachycardia (VT). Hypotension is less common with the aqueous solution.

Atropine

Atropine accelerates sinus and atrial pacemakers by blocking the parasympathetic response. It may also increase AV conduction. Small doses (<100 mcg) may cause paradoxical bradycardia.

Glucose

Neonatal, child and adult data show that both hyper- and hypoglycaemia are associated with poor outcome after cardiopulmonary arrest, but it is uncertain if this is causative or merely an association. Check blood or plasma glucose concentration and monitor closely in any ill or injured child, including after cardiac arrest. Do not give glucose-containing fluids during CPR unless hypoglycaemia is present. Avoid hyper- and hypoglycaemia following return of spontaneous circulation (ROSC).

Magnesium

There is no evidence for giving magnesium routinely during cardiopulmonary arrest. Magnesium treatment is indicated in the child with documented hypomagnesaemia or with torsades de pointes regardless of the cause.

Sodium bicarbonate

Giving sodium bicarbonate routinely during cardiopulmonary arrest and CPR or after ROSC is not recommended. After effective ventilation and chest compressions have been achieved and adrenaline given, sodium bicarbonate may be considered for the child who has had a prolonged cardiopulmonary arrest and severe metabolic acidosis. Sodium bicarbonate may also be considered in cases of haemodynamic instability and co-existing hyperkalaemia, or in the management of tricyclic overdose. Excessive quantities of sodium bicarbonate may impair tissue oxygen delivery, produce hypokalaemia, hypernatraemia, hyperosmolality and inactivate catecholamines.

Lidocaine

Lidocaine is less effective than amiodarone for defibrillation-resistant VF/pulseless VT in adults and therefore is not the first-line treatment in defibrillation-resistant VF/pulseless VT in children.

Procainamide

Procainamide slows intra-atrial conduction and prolongs the QRS and QT intervals; it can be used in SVT or VT resistant to other medications in the haemodynamically stable child.

However, paediatric data are sparse and procainamide should be used cautiously with careful monitoring.

Vasopressin

There is currently insufficient evidence to recommend the routine use of vasopressin in the child with cardiopulmonary arrest.

Defibrillators

Defibrillators are either automatically (such as the AED) or manually operated, and may be capable of delivering either monophasic or biphasic shocks. Manual defibrillators capable of delivering the full energy requirements from neonates upwards must be available within hospitals and in other healthcare facilities caring for children at risk of cardiopulmonary arrest. Automated external defibrillators are preset for all variables including the energy dose.

Pad/paddle size for defibrillation

The largest possible available paddles should be chosen to provide good contact with the chest wall. The ideal size is unknown but there should be good separation between the pads.

Recommended sizes are:

- 4.5 cm diameter for infants and children weighing <10 kg.
- 8–12 cm diameter for children >10 kg (older than 1 y).

To decrease skin and thoracic impedance, an electrically conducting interface is required between the skin and the paddles. Preformed gel pads or self-adhesive defibrillation electrodes are effective. Do not use saline-soaked gauze, alcohol-soaked gauze/pads or ultrasound gel.

Position of the paddles (Figure 5.8)

Apply the paddles firmly to the bare chest in the anterolateral position, one paddle placed below the right clavicle and the other in the left axilla. If the paddles are too large, and there is a danger of the charge arcing across the paddles, one should be placed on the upper back, below the left scapula, and the other on the front, to the left of the sternum. This is known as the anteroposterior position.

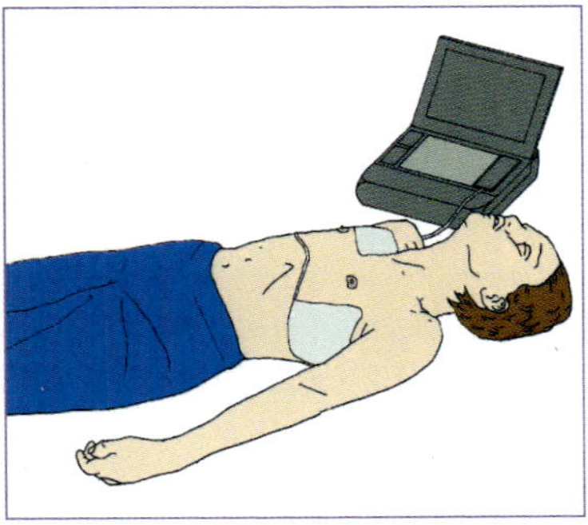

Figure 5.8. Paddle positions for defibrillation – child. © ERC 2005.

Optimal paddle force

To decrease transthoracic impedance during defibrillation, apply a force of 3 kg for children weighing <10 kg and 5 kg for larger children.

Energy dose in children

The ideal energy dose for safe and effective defibrillation is unknown. Biphasic shocks are at least as effective and produce less post-shock myocardial dysfunction than monophasic shocks. Doses larger than 4 J kg^{-1} (as much as 9 J kg^{-1}) have defibrillated children effectively with negligible side-effects. When using a manual defibrillator, use 4 J kg^{-1} (biphasic or monophasic waveform) for the first and subsequent shocks.

If no manual defibrillator is available, use an AED that can recognise paediatric shockable rhythms. This AED should be equipped with a dose attenuator which decreases the delivered energy to a lower dose more suitable for children aged 1–8 y (50–75 J). If such an AED is not available, in an emergency use a standard AED and the preset adult energy levels. For children weighing more than 25 kg (above 8 y), use a standard AED with standard paddles. There is currently insufficient evidence to support a recommendation for or against the use of AEDs in children less than 1 y.

Management of cardiopulmonary arrest (Figure 5.9)

A B C **Commence and continue with basic life support.**

A and B **Oxygenate and ventilate with BMV.**

- Provide positive pressure ventilation with a high inspired oxygen concentration.
- Give five rescue breaths followed by external chest compression and positive pressure ventilation in the ratio of 15:2 (lone rescuer may use 30:2).
- Avoid rescuer fatigue by changing the rescuer performing chest compressions frequently.
- Establish cardiac monitoring.

C **Assess cardiac rhythm and signs of circulation.**

(± check for a central pulse for no more than 10 s.)

Asystole, pulseless electrical activity (PEA) – non-shockable

- Give adrenaline IV or IO (10 mcg kg^{-1}) and repeat every 3–5 min.
- If no vascular access is available and a tracheal tube is in situ give adrenaline (100 mcg kg^{-1}) via this route until IV/IO access is obtained.
- Identify and treat any reversible causes (4Hs and 4Ts).

VF/ pulseless VT – shockable

- Attempt defibrillation immediately (4 J kg^{-1} for all shocks).
- Resume CPR as soon as possible.
- After 2 min, check the cardiac rhythm on the monitor.
- Give second shock if still in VF/pulseless VT.
- Immediately resume CPR for 2 min and check monitor; if no change, give adrenaline followed immediately by a third shock.
- Give CPR for 2 min.
- Give amiodarone if still in VF/pulseless VT followed immediately by a fourth shock.
- Give adrenaline every 3–5 min during CPR.

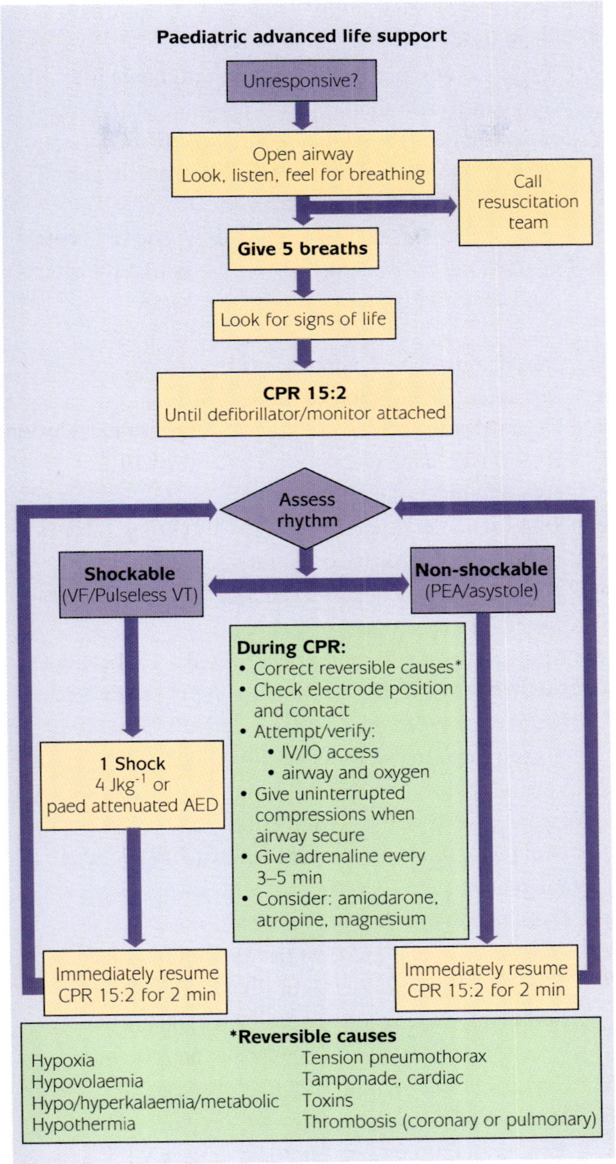

Figure 5.9. Paediatric advanced life support algorithm.

- If the child remains in VF/pulseless VT, continue to alternate shocks with 2 min of CPR.
- If signs of life become evident, check the monitor for an organised rhythm; if this is present check for a central pulse.
- Identify and treat any reversible causes (4Hs and 4Ts).
- If defibrillation was successful but VF/pulseless VT recurs, resume CPR, give amiodarone and defibrillate again at the dose that was effective previously. Start a continuous infusion of amiodarone.

Reversible causes of cardiac arrest (4Hs and 4Ts)

- Hypoxia.
- Hypovolaemia.
- Hyper/hypokalaemia.
- Hypothermia.
- Tension pneumothorax.
- Tamponade (coronary or pulmonary).
- Toxic/therapeutic disturbances.
- Thrombosis (coronary or pulmonary).

Arrhythmias

Unstable arrhythmias

Check the central pulse of any child with an arrhythmia; if the pulse is absent, proceed to treating the child as being in cardiopulmonary arrest. If the child has a central pulse, evaluate his haemodynamic status. Whenever the haemodynamic status is compromised, the first steps are:

1. Open the airway.
2. Assist ventilation and give oxygen.
3. Attach ECG monitor or defibrillator and assess the cardiac rhythm.
4. Evaluate if the rhythm is slow or fast for the child's age.
5. Evaluate if the rhythm is regular or irregular.
6. Measure QRS complex (narrow complexes: <0.08 s duration; large complexes: >0.08 s).
7. The treatment options are dependent on the child's haemodynamic stability.

Bradycardia

Bradycardia is caused commonly by hypoxia, acidosis and severe hypotension; it may progress to cardiopulmonary arrest. Give 100% oxygen, and positive pressure ventilation if required, to any child presenting with bradyarrhythmia and circulatory failure.

If a poorly perfused child has a heart rate <60 beats min^{-1}, and it does not respond rapidly to ventilation with oxygen, start chest compressions and give adrenaline. If the bradycardia is caused by vagal stimulation, provide ventilation with 100% oxygen and give atropine, before giving adrenaline.

A cardiac pacemaker is useful only in cases of AV block or sinus node dysfunction unresponsive to oxygenation, ventilation, chest compressions and other medications; the pacemaker is not effective in asystole or arrhythmias caused by hypoxia or ischaemia.

Tachycardia

Narrow complex tachycardia

If supraventricular tachycardia (SVT) is the likely rhythm, vagal manoeuvres (Valsalva or diving reflex) may be used in haemodynamically stable children. They can be used in unstable children if they do not delay chemical or electrical cardioversion. If the child is too haemodynamically unstable, omit vagal manoeuvres and attempt electrical cardioversion immediately. Adenosine is usually effective in converting SVT into sinus rhythm.

Electrical cardioversion (synchronised with R wave) is indicated in the haemodynamically compromised child, in whom vascular access is not available, or in whom adenosine has failed to convert the rhythm. The first energy dose for electrical cardioversion of SVT is 0.5–1 J kg^{-1} and the second dose is 2 J kg^{-1}. If unsuccessful, give amiodarone or procainamide under guidance from a paediatric cardiologist or intensivist before the third attempt.

Amiodarone has been shown to be effective in the treatment of SVT in several paediatric studies. If the child is haemodynamically stable, early consultation with an expert is recommended before giving amiodarone.

Wide complex tachycardia

In children, wide QRS complex tachycardia is more likely to be supraventricular than ventricular in origin. Wide QRS complex tachycardia, although uncommon, must be considered to be VT in haemodynamically unstable children until proven otherwise. Ventricular tachycardia occurs most often in the child with underlying heart disease (e.g. after cardiac surgery, cardiomyopathy, myocarditis, electrolyte disorders, prolonged QT interval, central intracardiac catheter). Synchronised cardioversion is the treatment of choice for unstable VT with a pulse. Consider anti-arrhythmic therapy if a second cardioversion dose is unsuccessful or if VT recurs. Amiodarone has been shown to be safe and effective in treating paediatric arrhythmias.

Stable arrhythmias

Contact an expert before initiating therapy, whilst maintaining the child's ABC. Depending on the child's clinical history, presentation and ECG diagnosis, a child with stable, wide QRS complex tachycardia may be treated for SVT and be given vagal manoeuvres or adenosine. Otherwise, consider amiodarone as a treatment option; similarly, consider amiodarone if the diagnosis of VT is confirmed by ECG. Procainamide may also be considered in stable SVT refractory to vagal manoeuvres and adenosine as well as in stable VT. Do not give procainamide with amiodarone.

Post-arrest management

Temperature control and management

Hypothermia is common in the child following cardiopulmonary resuscitation. Central hypothermia (32–34°C) may be beneficial, whereas fever may be detrimental to the injured brain of survivors. Although there are no paediatric studies, mild hypothermia has an acceptable safety profile in adults and neonates; it could increase the number of neurologically intact survivors.

A child who regains a spontaneous circulation but remains comatose after cardiopulmonary arrest may benefit from being cooled to a core temperature of 32–34°C for 12–24 h. The successfully resuscitated child with hypothermia and ROSC should not be actively re-warmed unless the core temperature is below 32°C. The optimum target temperature, rate of cooling, duration of hypothermia and rate of rewarming after deliberate cooling have yet to be determined; currently, no specific protocol for children can be recommended. Following a period of mild hypothermia, rewarm the child slowly at 0.25–0.5°C h^{-1}.

Fever is common following cardiopulmonary resuscitation; it is associated with a poor neurological outcome, the risk increasing for each degree of body temperature greater than 37°C. There are limited experimental data suggesting that the treatment of fever with antipyretics and/or physical cooling reduces neuronal damage. Antipyretics and accepted drugs to treat fever are safe; therefore, use them to treat fever aggressively.

Prognosis of cardiopulmonary arrest

There are no simple guidelines to determine when resuscitative efforts become futile.

After 20 min of resuscitation the team leader of the resuscitation team should consider whether or not to stop. The relevant considerations in the decision to continue the resuscitation include the cause of arrest, pre-existing conditions, whether the arrest was witnessed, the duration of untreated cardiopulmonary arrest ('no flow'), the effectiveness and duration of CPR ('low flow'), the promptness of extracorporeal life support for a reversible disease process and associated special circumstances (e.g. icy water drowning, exposure to toxic drugs).

Parental presence

The majority of parents would like to be present during resuscitation and when any procedure is carried out on their child. Parents witnessing their child's resuscitation can see that everything possible has been attempted. Families who were present at their child's death showed less anxiety and depression, better adjustment and had an improved grieving process when assessed several months later. Parental presence in the resuscitation room may help healthcare providers maintain their professional behaviour, whilst helping them to see the child as a human being and a family member.

Family presence guidelines

A dedicated member of the resuscitation team should be present with the parents to explain the process in an empathetic manner, ensuring that the parents do not interfere with or distract the resuscitation. If the presence of the parents is impeding the progress of the resuscitation, they should be sensitively asked to leave. When appropriate, physical contact with the child should be allowed and, wherever possible, the parents should be allowed to be with their dying child at the final moment.

The leader of the resuscitation team, not the parents, will decide when to stop the resuscitation; this should be expressed with sensitivity and understanding. After the event, the team should be debriefed, to enable any concerns to be expressed and for the team to reflect on their clinical practice in a supportive environment.

Resuscitation of babies at birth

Introduction

During normal labour, respiratory gas exchange at the placenta ceases during the 60–90 s of the average uterine contraction. During the second stage of labour, these contractions are occurring perhaps four times every 10 min. Passage through the birth canal is a hypoxic experience for the human fetus. Though most babies tolerate this well, some do not and these few may require help to establish normal breathing at delivery. Newborn life support is intended to provide this help and it comprises the following elements: drying and covering the newborn baby to conserve heat, assessing the need for any intervention, airway opening, lung aeration, rescue breathing, chest compressions and, very rarely, the administration of drugs.

The newborn is uniquely adapted to withstand the hypoxic experience of birth (see below). When a baby is in difficulty at birth the single most important intervention is to aerate the lungs effectively. Almost all babies will respond once the lungs have been aerated. The few that do not will probably respond to a brief period of chest compressions, but only if their lungs have first been aerated successfully, leaving a tiny minority who might possibly respond to drugs.

Physiology

If subjected to continuing hypoxia in utero, the fetus will start making breathing movements but will eventually stop this as the neural centres controlling breathing cease to function due to lack of oxygen. The fetus then enters a period known as 'primary' apnoea.

By this time the oxygen content of the fetal blood is minimal and the heart rate rapidly falls to about half its normal rate as it reverts to anaerobic metabolism – a less fuel-efficient mechanism. However, the circulation to vital organs is maintained, with little loss of blood pressure, by shutting down blood flow to non-vital areas.

If the insult continues then, after a variable period of time, primitive spinal centres, released from suppression by the higher breathing centres, initiate shuddering whole body gasps at a rate of about 12 min^{-1}. If these gasps fail to aerate the lungs then they also fade away and the fetus enters a period known as 'secondary' or 'terminal' apnoea.

Up until now, the circulation is maintained but, as terminal apnoea progresses, the rapidly deteriorating biochemical milieu increasingly impairs cardiac function, which eventually fails and, without effective intervention, the baby dies. The whole process probably takes almost 20 min in the term newborn human baby.

The fetus is thus appropriately adapted in preparation for the anoxic events of normal labour. An effective circulation can be maintained throughout the period of primary apnoea, through the gasping phase and even for a while after the onset of terminal apnoea. Should the lungs be aerated during this period then the circulation is still capable of picking up oxygen from the lungs and returning this to the heart.

Once one is aware of this sequence of events it becomes clear that the most urgent requirement of any asphyxiated baby at birth is that the lungs should be aerated effectively. Then, provided the baby's circulation is sufficiently intact, oxygenated blood will be conveyed from the aerated lungs to the heart, which in turn will respond by increasing in rate and by distributing oxygenated blood to the brain. Following this the neural centres responsible for normal breathing will, in many instances, function once again and the baby will recover.

Merely aerating the lungs is sufficient in the vast majority of cases. However, though lung aeration is still vital, in a few cases cardiac function will have deteriorated such that the circulation is inadequate and it cannot convey oxygenated blood from the aerated lungs to the heart, in which case a brief period of chest compression may be needed to achieve this. In a very small number of cases lung aeration and chest compression will not be sufficient, in which case drugs may help to restore the circulation. The outlook in this last group is poor.

Preparation

Resuscitation at birth is more likely to be needed by babies with intrapartum evidence of significant fetal compromise, babies delivering before 35 weeks gestation, babies delivering vaginally by the breech, and multiple pregnancies.

Although it is often possible to predict the need for resuscitation before a baby is born, this is not always the case. Therefore, personnel trained in newborn life support should be easily available at every delivery and, should there be any need for resuscitation, the care of the baby should be their sole responsibility.

One person experienced in tracheal intubation of the newborn should also be easily available for normal low-risk deliveries and, ideally, in attendance for deliveries associated with a high risk for neonatal resuscitation.

Local guidelines indicating who should attend deliveries should be developed based on current practice and clinical audit.

An organised educational programme in the standards and skills required for resuscitation of the newborn is therefore essential for any institution in which deliveries occur.

Equipment and environment

Resuscitation should ideally take place in a warm, well-lit, draught-free area with a flat resuscitation surface placed below a radiant heater, with other resuscitation equipment immediately available. All equipment must be checked daily.

When a birth takes place in a non-designated delivery area, the recommended minimum set of equipment includes a device for safe assisted lung aeration of an appropriate size for the newborn, warm dry towels and blankets, a clean (sterile) instrument for cutting the umbilical cord and clean gloves for the attendant. It may also be helpful to have a suction device with a suitably sized suction catheter and a tongue depressor (or laryngoscope) to enable the oropharynx to be examined.

Temperature control

Naked, wet, newborn babies cannot maintain their body temperature even in a room that feels comfortably warm for adults. Compromised babies are particularly vulnerable. Exposure of the newborn to cold stress will lower arterial oxygen tension and increase metabolic acidosis. Prevent heat loss by:

- Drying the term baby immediately after delivery. Cover the head and body of the baby, apart from the face, with a warm towel to prevent further heat loss. Alternatively, place the baby skin to skin with mother and cover both with a towel.
- If the baby needs resuscitation then place the baby on a warm surface under a preheated radiant warmer.
- In very preterm babies (especially below 28 weeks) drying and wrapping may not be sufficient. A more effective method is to cover the head and body of the

baby (apart from the face) with plastic wrapping, without drying the baby beforehand, and then to place the baby so covered under radiant heat.

Initial assessment

Respiratory activity

Check whether the baby is breathing. If so, evaluate the rate, depth and symmetry of respiration, together with any abnormal breathing pattern such as gasping or grunting.

Heart rate

This is best evaluated by listening to the apex beat with a stethoscope. Feeling the pulse in the base of the umbilical cord is often effective but can be misleading; cord pulsation is only reliable if found to be more than 100 beats min^{-1}.

Colour

A healthy baby is born blue but becomes pink within 30 s of the onset of effective breathing. Observe whether the baby is centrally pink, cyanosed or pale. Peripheral cyanosis is common and does not, by itself, indicate hypoxaemia.

Tone

A very floppy baby is likely to be unconscious and is likely to need respiratory support.

Classification according to initial assessment

On the basis of the initial assessment, the babies can usually be divided into four groups:

1. Vigorous breathing or crying.
- Good tone.
- Rapidly becoming pink.
- Heart rate greater than 100 min^{-1}.

This baby requires no intervention other than drying, wrapping in a warm towel and, where appropriate, handing to the mother. The baby will remain warm through skin-to-skin contact with mother under a cover, and may be put to the breast at this stage.

2. Breathing inadequately or apnoeic.
- Remaining centrally blue.
- Normal or reduced tone.
- Heart rate less than 100 min^{-1}.

This baby may respond to tactile stimulation and/or facial oxygen but may need mask inflation.

3. Breathing inadequately or apnoeic.
- Blue or pale.
- Floppy.
- Heart rate less than 100 min^{-1}.

This baby may improve with mask inflation but may also require chest compressions.

4. Breathing inadequately or apnoeic.
- Pale.
- Floppy.
- No detectable heart rate.

This baby will require immediate airway control, lung inflation and ventilation. Once this has been accomplished successfully, the baby may also need chest compressions, and perhaps drugs.

There remains a very rare group of babies who, though breathing adequately and with a good heart rate, remain blue. This group includes a range of possible diagnoses such as diaphragmatic hernia, surfactant deficiency, congenital pneumonia, pneumothorax, or cyanotic congenital heart disease.

Newborn life support (Figure 5.10)

Commence newborn life support if the baby has failed to establish adequate regular normal breathing within a minute or two of birth, or if the baby has a heart rate of less than 100 min^{-1}. Opening the airway and aerating the lungs is usually all that is necessary. Furthermore, more complex interventions will be futile unless these first two steps have been completed successfully.

The baby should be on his or her back with the head in a neutral position (Figure 5.11). A 2 cm thickness of the blanket or towel placed under the baby's shoulder may be

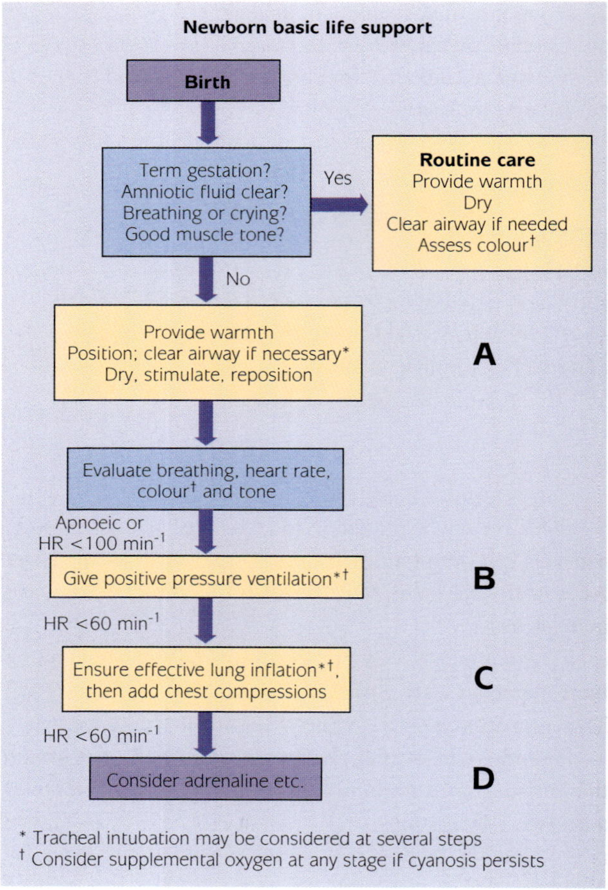

Figure 5.10. Algorithm for resuscitation of the newborn.

helpful in maintaining proper head position. In floppy babies application of jaw thrust or an appropriately sized oropharyngeal airway may be helpful in opening the airway.

Suction is needed only if there is particulate matter or blood obstructing the airway. Aggressive pharyngeal suction can delay the onset of spontaneous breathing and cause laryngeal spasm and vagal bradycardia. The presence of thick meconium in a non-vigorous baby is the only indication for considering immediate suction. If suction is required it is best done under direct vision. Connect a 12–14 FG suction catheter, or a Yankauer sucker, to a suction source with a negative pressure not exceeding 100 mmHg.

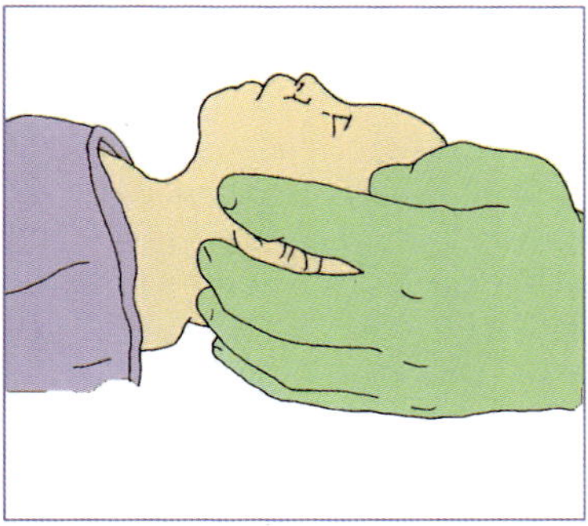

Figure 5.11. Newborn head in neutral position.
© Resuscitation Council UK 2005.

There is currently insufficient evidence to specify the concentration of oxygen to be used when starting resuscitation. After initial steps at birth, if respiratory efforts are absent or inadequate, lung aeration is the priority (Figure 5.12). The primary measure of adequate initial lung inflation is a prompt improvement in heart rate; assess chest wall movement if heart rate does not improve.

For the first few breaths it may be helpful to maintain the initial inflation pressure for 2–3 s. This will help lung aeration. Most babies needing resuscitation at birth will respond with a rapid increase in heart rate within 30 seconds of lung inflation. If the heart rate increases but the baby is not breathing adequately, continue ventilation at a rate of about 30 breaths min^{-1}, allowing approximately 1 s for each inflation, until there is adequate spontaneous breathing.

Adequate passive ventilation is usually indicated by either a rapidly increasing heart rate or a heart rate that is maintained above 100 beats min^{-1}. If the baby does not respond in this way the most likely reason is inadequate airway control or ventilation. Look for passive chest movement in time with inflation efforts; if these are present then lung aeration has been achieved. If these are absent then airway control and lung aeration have not been confirmed. Without adequate lung aeration chest compressions will be ineffective; therefore, confirm lung aeration before progressing to circulatory support.

Some practitioners will ensure lung aeration by tracheal intubation, but this requires training and experience to be achieved effectively. If this skill is not available and the heart rate is decreasing, re-evaluate airway position and deliver aeration breaths while summoning a colleague with intubation skills.

Continue ventilatory support until the baby has established normal regular breathing.

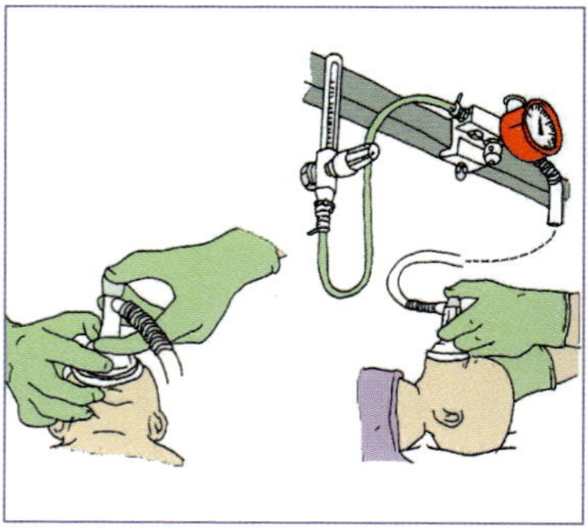

Figure 5.12. Airway and ventilation – newborn. © Resuscitation Council UK 2005.

Circulatory support

Circulatory support with chest compressions is effective only if the lungs have been successfully inflated first. Give chest compressions if the heart rate is less than 60 beats min^{-1} despite adequate ventilation (Figure 5.13).

The optimal technique is to place the two thumbs side by side over the lower third of the sternum with the fingers encircling the torso and supporting the back. Briskly compress the lower third of the sternum to a depth of approximately one-third of the anterior–posterior diameter of the chest. Try not to lift the thumbs off the sternum during the relaxation phase, but allow the chest wall to return to its relaxed position between compressions.

Use a 3:1 ratio of compressions to ventilations, aiming to achieve approximately 120 events per minute, i.e. approximately 90 compressions and 30 breaths. However, the quality of the compressions and breaths are more important than the rate.

Check the heart rate after about 30 s and periodically thereafter. Discontinue chest compressions when the spontaneous heart rate is faster then 60 beats min^{-1}.

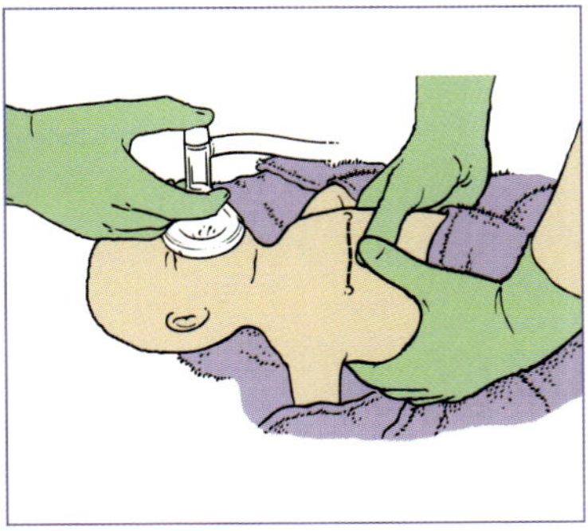

Figure 5.13. Ventilation and chest compression – newborn. © Resuscitation Council UK 2005.

Drugs

Drugs are rarely indicated in resuscitation of the newly born infant. Bradycardia in the newborn infant is usually caused by inadequate lung inflation or profound hypoxia, and establishing adequate ventilation is the most important step to correct it.

However, if the heart rate remains less than 60 beats min^{-1} despite adequate ventilation and chest compressions, drugs may be needed. These drugs are presumed to exert their effect by their action on the heart and are being given because cardiac function is inadequate. It is therefore necessary to give them as close to the heart as possible, ideally via a rapidly inserted umbilical venous catheter (Figure 5.14).

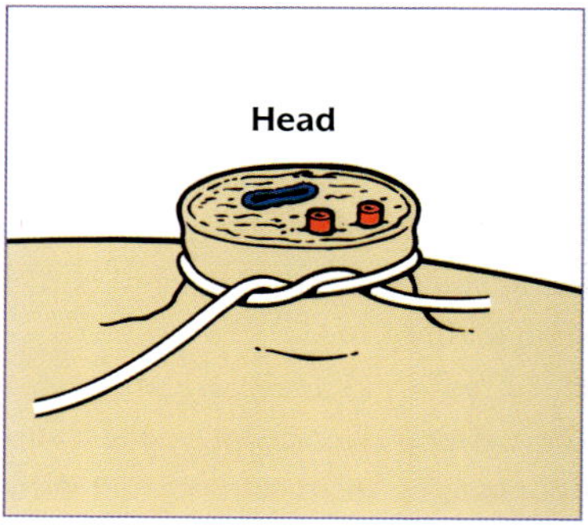

Figure 5.14. Newborn umbilical cord showing the position of the arteries and vein. © Resuscitation Council UK 2005.

Adrenaline

Despite the lack of human data it is reasonable to continue to use adrenaline when adequate ventilation and chest compressions have failed to increase the heart rate above 60 beats min^{-1}. Use the intravenous route as soon as venous access is established. The recommended intravenous dose is 10–30 mcg kg^{-1}.

The tracheal route is not recommended but if it is used, it is highly likely that doses of 30 mcg kg^{-1} or less are ineffective. Consider a higher dose (up to 100 mcg kg^{-1}), but the safety of these higher tracheal doses has not been studied. Do not give high doses intravenously.

Bicarbonate

If effective spontaneous cardiac output is not restored despite adequate ventilation and adequate chest compressions, reversing intracardiac acidosis may improve myocardial function and achieve a spontaneous circulation. Give 1–2 mmol kg^{-1} intravenously.

Fluids

Consider volume expansion when there has been suspected blood loss or the infant appears to be in shock (pale, poor perfusion, weak pulse) and has not responded adequately to other resuscitative measures. In the absence of suitable blood (i.e. irradiated and leucocyte-depleted group O Rh-negative blood) isotonic crystalloid rather than albumin is the solution of choice for restoring intravascular volume in the delivery room. Give a bolus of 10–20 ml kg^{-1}.

Stopping resuscitation

Local and national committees will determine the indications for stopping resuscitation. However, data from infants without signs of life from birth lasting at least 10 min or longer show either high mortality or severe neurodevelopmental disability. After 10 min of continuous and adequate resuscitation efforts, discontinuation of resuscitation may be justified if there are no signs of life.

Communication with the parents

It is vitally important that the team caring for the newborn baby informs the parents of the baby's progress. At delivery adhere to the routine local plan and, if possible, hand the baby to the mother at the earliest opportunity. If resuscitation is required, inform the parents of the procedures being undertaken and why they are required.

Decisions to discontinue resuscitation ideally should involve senior paediatric staff. Whenever possible, the decision to attempt resuscitation of an extremely preterm baby should be taken in close consultation with the parents and senior paediatric and obstetric staff. Where a difficulty has been foreseen, for example in the case of severe congenital malformation, the options and prognosis should be discussed with the parents, midwives, obstetricians and birth attendants before delivery.

All discussions and decisions should be carefully recorded in the mother's notes prior to delivery and also in the baby's records after birth.

Specific questions addressed at the 2005 Consensus Conference

Maintaining normal temperature in preterm infants

Placing the preterm baby under radiant heat and then covering the baby with food-grade plastic wrapping without drying significantly improves temperature on admission to intensive care compared with traditional techniques. The baby's temperature must be monitored closely because of the small, but described, risk of hyperthermia with this technique. All resuscitation procedures, including intubation, chest compression and insertion of lines, can be achieved with the plastic cover in place.

Infants born to febrile mothers have been reported to have a higher incidence of perinatal respiratory depression, neonatal seizures, early mortality and cerebral palsy. Animal studies indicate that hyperthermia during or following ischaemia is associated with a progression of cerebral injury. Hyperthermia should be avoided.

Meconium

Five years ago a large randomised controlled study showed that attempting to intubate and aspirate inhaled meconium from the tracheas of vigorous infants at birth was not beneficial. A more recent large multicentre randomised controlled study has now shown that suctioning meconium from the baby's nose and mouth before delivery of the baby's chest (intrapartum suctioning) does not reduce the incidence or severity of meconium aspiration syndrome. Intrapartum suctioning is therefore no longer recommended.

Intubation and suction of meconium from the trachea of non-vigorous infants born through meconium-stained liquor is still recommended.

Air or 100% oxygen

Several studies in recent years have raised concerns about the potential adverse effects of 100% oxygen on respiratory physiology, cerebral circulation and potential tissue damage from oxygen free radicals. There are also concerns about tissue damage from oxygen deprivation during and following asphyxia.

At present, the standard approach to resuscitation is to use 100% oxygen. Some clinicians may elect to start resuscitation with an oxygen concentration less than 100%, including some who may start with air. Evidence suggests that this approach may be reasonable. However, where possible, supplemental oxygen should be available for use should there be no rapid improvement following successful lung aeration. If supplemental oxygen is not readily available, ventilate the lungs with air. Supplemental oxygen is recommended for babies who are breathing but have central cyanosis.

Healthy term newborn babies may take more than 10 min to achieve a preductal oxygen saturation above 95% following delivery. However, monitoring of oxygen saturation in resuscitation may be helpful in avoiding hyperoxia, especially in preterm infants.

Initial breaths and assisted ventilation

In term infants, spontaneous or assisted initial inflations create a functional residual capacity (FRC). The optimum pressure, inflation time and flow required to establish an effective FRC have not been determined. Average initial peak inflating pressures of 30–40 cm H_2O (inflation time undefined) usually ventilate unresponsive term infants successfully. Assisted ventilation rates of 30–60 breaths min^{-1} are used commonly, but the relative efficacy of various rates has not been investigated.

The primary measure of adequate initial lung aeration is prompt increase in heart rate; assess passive chest wall movement if heart rate does not increase. The initial peak inflating pressures needed are variable and unpredictable and should be individualised to achieve an increase in heart rate or movement of the chest with each breath. Where pressure is being monitored, an initial inflation pressure of 20 cm H_2O may be effective, but 30–40 cm H_2O or higher may be required in some term babies. If pressure is not being monitored but merely limited by a non-adjustable 'blow-off' valve, use the minimum inflation pressure required to achieve an increase in heart rate. There is insufficient evidence to recommend an optimum inflation time. In summary, provide artificial ventilation at 30–60 breaths min^{-1} to achieve or maintain a heart rate higher than 100 beats min^{-1} promptly.

Assisted ventilation of preterm infants

Animal studies show that preterm lungs are easily damaged by large volume inflations immediately after birth and that maintaining a positive end expiratory pressure (PEEP) immediately after birth protects against lung damage. Positive end expiratory pressure also improves lung compliance and gas exchange. Human case series show that most apnoeic preterm infants can be ventilated with an initial inflation pressure of 20–25 cm H_2O, though some infants appear to require a higher pressure.

When ventilating preterm infants, very obvious passive chest wall movement may indicate excessive tidal volumes and should be avoided. Monitoring of pressure may help to provide consistent inflations and avoid high pressures. If positive-pressure ventilation is required, an initial inflation pressure of 20–25 cm H_2O is adequate for most preterm infants. If a prompt increase in heart rate or chest movement is not obtained, higher pressures may be needed. If continued positive-pressure ventilation is required, PEEP may be beneficial. Continuous positive airway pressure (CPAP) in spontaneously breathing preterm infants following resuscitation may also be beneficial.

Devices

A self-inflating bag, a flow-inflating bag or a T-piece mechanical device, all designed to regulate or limit the pressure applied to the airway, can be used to ventilate a newborn.

The blow-off valves of self-inflating bags are flow-dependent and pressures generated by vigorous squeezing may exceed the value specified by the manufacturer. Target inflation pressures and long inspiratory times are achieved more consistently in mechanical models when using T-piece devices than when using bags, although the clinical implications are not clear. More training is required to provide an appropriate pressure using flow-inflating bags compared with self-inflating bags.

Laryngeal mask airways (LMAs) are effective for ventilating newly born near-term and full-term infants in the hands of experienced users. Case reports suggest that when bag-mask ventilation has been unsuccessful and tracheal intubation is unfeasible or unsuccessful, the LMA may provide effective ventilation. There is insufficient evidence to support the routine use of the LMA as the primary airway device for resuscitation at birth. There are also reservations concerning its effectiveness in the following situations:

- When chest compressions are required.
- For very low birth weight (VLBW) babies.
- When the amniotic fluid is meconium-stained.

Confirming tracheal tube placement

The use and timing of tracheal intubation will depend on the skill and experience of the available resuscitators.

Following tracheal intubation and intermittent positive pressure, a prompt increase in heart rate is the best indicator that the tube is in the tracheobronchial tree. Detection of exhaled CO_2 in patients with adequate cardiac output confirms placement of the tube within the trachea, whereas failure to detect exhaled CO_2 strongly suggests oesophageal intubation. However, poor or absent pulmonary blood flow or tracheal obstruction may prevent detection of exhaled CO_2 despite correct tracheal tube placement.

Tracheal tube placement must be assessed visually during intubation and, in most cases, will be confirmed by a rapid increase in heart rate on ventilating via the tracheal tube. If the heart rate remains slow, incorrect tube placement is the most likely cause. Check tube placement either visually or by detection of exhaled CO_2.

See Table 5.2 for appropriate tube size and depth of insertion of the tracheal tube. Depth of insertion from the upper lip can be estimated from:

Insertion depth at lip (cm) = weight in kg + 6 cm

Table 5.2 Tracheal tube insertion

Weight (kg)	Gestation (week)	Tube size (mm ID)	Depth of insertion at upper lip (cm)
<1	<28	2.5	6.5–7
1–2	28–34	3.0	7–8
2–3	34–38	3.0/3.5	8–9
>3	>38	3.5/4.0	>9

Post-resuscitation care

Babies who have required resuscitation may deteriorate. Once adequate ventilation and circulation are established, the infant should be maintained in or transferred to an environment in which close monitoring and anticipatory care can be provided.

Glucose

The range of blood glucose concentration that is associated with the least brain injury following asphyxia and resuscitation cannot be defined based on available evidence. Infants who require significant resuscitation should be monitored and treated to maintain glucose in the normal range.

Induced hypothermia

There are insufficient data to recommend routine use of modest systemic or selective cerebral hypothermia following resuscitation of infants with suspected asphyxia. Further clinical trials are needed to determine which infants benefit most and which method of cooling is most effective.

Withholding or discontinuing resuscitation

Mortality and morbidity for newborns varies according to region and to availability of resources. Social science studies indicate that parents desire a larger role in decisions to resuscitate and to continue life support in severely compromised babies. There is considerable variability among providers about the benefits and disadvantages of aggressive therapies in such babies.

Withholding resuscitation

It is possible to identify conditions associated with high mortality and poor outcome, where withholding resuscitation may be considered reasonable, particularly when there has been the opportunity for discussion with parents.

A consistent and coordinated approach to individual cases by the obstetric and neonatal teams and the parents is an important goal. Withholding resuscitation and discontinuation of life-sustaining treatment during or following resuscitation are considered by many to be ethically equivalent and clinicians should not be hesitant to withdraw support when the possibility of functional survival is highly unlikely. The following guidelines must be interpreted according to current regional outcomes:

- Where gestation, birth weight and/or congenital anomalies are associated with almost certain early death, and unacceptably high morbidity is likely among the rare survivors, resuscitation is not indicated. Examples from the published literature include: extreme prematurity (gestational age <23 weeks and/or birth weight <400 g), and anomalies such as anencephaly and confirmed Trisomy 13 or 18.
- Resuscitation is nearly always indicated in conditions associated with a high survival rate and acceptable morbidity. This will generally include babies with gestational age of 25 weeks or above (unless there is evidence of fetal compromise such as intrauterine infection or hypoxia–ischaemia) and those with most congenital malformations.
- In conditions associated with uncertain prognosis, where survival is unlikely and associated with a relatively high rate of morbidity, and where the anticipated burden to the child is high, parental desires regarding resuscitation should be supported.

Withdrawing resuscitation efforts

Data from infants without signs of life from birth, lasting at least 10 min or longer, show either high mortality or severe neurodevelopmental disability. After 10 min of uninterrupted and adequate resuscitation efforts, discontinuation of resuscitation may be justified if there are no signs of life.

Further reading

1. International Liaison Committee on Resuscitation. 2005 International Consensus on Cardiopulmonary Resuscitation and Emergency Cardiovascular Care Science with Treatment Recommendations. Resuscitation 2005;67:271–303.
2. European Resuscitation Council. European Resuscitation Council guidelines for resuscitation 2005. Resuscitation 2005;67(Suppl 1):S97–133.

Chapter 6
Cardiac arrest in special circumstances

Jasmeet Soar, Charles D Deakin, Jerry P Nolan, Gamal Abbas, Annette Alfonzo, Anthony Handley, David Lockey, Gavin D Perkins and Karl Thies

1. Life-threatening electrolyte disorders

- Electrolyte abnormalities can cause arrhythmias or cardiopulmonary arrest.
- Potassium disorders, particularly hyperkalaemia, are the most common.
- If suspected start treatment before laboratory results available.

Potassium disorders

Hyperkalaemia

Recognition

- Serum potassium above 5.5 mmol l^{-1}. Severe hyperkalaemia is a serum potassium above 6.5 mmol l^{-1}.
- Usually due to increased K^+ release from cells or impaired excretion by kidneys.
- Causes include renal failure, drugs, tissue breakdown (rhabdomyolysis, tumour lysis, haemolysis), metabolic acidosis, endocrine disorders (Addison's disease), hyperkalaemic periodic paralysis or diet.
- Presentation: weakness, flaccid paralysis, paraesthesia or depressed reflexes, ECG abnormalities, arrhythmias, cardiopulmonary arrest or sudden death.
- ECG changes include: first degree heart block, flattened or absent P waves, tall peaked (tented) T waves, widened QRS, bradycardia, VT, VF, PEA, asystole.

Treatment of hyperkalaemia

- **Patient not in cardiac arrest**

If hypovolaemic, give fluid to enhance urinary potassium loss. Values for classification are an approximate guide.

Mild elevation (5.5–6 mmol l^{-1}), remove K^+ from the body with:

1. Potassium exchange resins – calcium resonium 15–30 g **or** sodium polystyrene sulphonate (Kayexalate) 15–30 g in 50–100 ml of 20% sorbitol. Give orally or by retention enema (onset in 1–3 h; maximal effect at 6 h).
2. Diuretics – furosemide 1 mg kg^{-1} IV slowly (onset with the diuresis).
3. Dialysis – haemodialysis more efficient than peritoneal dialysis at removing potassium (immediate onset; 25–30 mmol K^+ h^{-1} removed with haemodialysis).

Moderate elevation (6–6.5 mmol l^{-1}) without ECG changes, shift K^+ intracellularly with:

1. Dextrose/insulin – 10 units short-acting insulin and 50 g glucose IV over 15–30 min (monitor blood glucose). Use in addition to removal strategies above.

Severe elevation (≥6.5 mmol l^{-1}) *without* ECG changes, shift K^+ intracellularly with:

1. Salbutamol – 5 mg nebulised. Several doses may be required.
2. Sodium bicarbonate – 50 mmol IV over 5 min if metabolic acidosis. Bicarbonate alone is less effective than glucose plus insulin or nebulised salbutamol.

Use multiple shifting agents in addition to removal strategies above.

Severe elevation (≥6.5 mmol/l) *with* toxic ECG changes, protect the heart **first** with:

1. Calcium chloride – 10 ml 10% calcium chloride IV over 2–5 min to antagonise the toxic effects of hyperkalaemia at the myocardial cell membrane. This lowers the risk of VF, but does not lower serum potassium.

Use in addition to potassium removal and shifting strategies stated above.

- **Patient in cardiac arrest**

Protect the heart first; then use shifting and removal strategies:

1. Calcium chloride – 10 ml 10% calcium chloride IV rapid injection to antagonise the toxic effects of hyperkalaemia at the myocardial cell membrane.
2. Sodium bicarbonate – 50 mmol IV rapid injection (if severe acidosis or renal failure).
3. Dextrose/insulin – 10 units short-acting insulin and 50 g glucose IV by rapid injection.
4. Haemodialysis – consider this for cardiac arrest induced by hyperkalaemia which is resistant to medical treatment.

Hypokalaemia

Recognition

- Defined as a serum potassium <3.5 mmol l^{-1}. Severe hypokalaemia is defined as a K^+ <2.5 mmol l^{-1}.
- Causes include diarrhoea, drugs, renal losses, endocrine disorders (Cushing's syndrome, hyperaldosteronism), metabolic alkalosis, magnesium depletion and poor dietary intake.
- Nerves and muscles predominantly affected, causing fatigue, weakness, leg cramps, constipation. If rhabdomyolysis, ascending paralysis and respiratory difficulties.

Treatment of hypokalemia

- Gradual replacement of potassium is preferable.
- Maximum IV dose of potassium is 20 mmol h^{-1}.
- Consider more rapid administration if cardiac arrest is imminent.
- ECG monitoring essential. Titrate dose based on serial K^+ measurements.
- Repletion of magnesium stores for more rapid correction of hypokalaemia.

Calcium and magnesium disorders

The recognition and management of calcium and magnesium disorders is summarised in Table 6.1.

2. Poisoning

- Use an ABCDE approach to prevent cardiorespiratory arrest whilst awaiting drug elimination.

Table 6.1 Calcium and magnesium disorders

Disorder	Causes	Presentation
Hypercalcaemia $[Ca^{2+}]$ >2.6 mmol l^{-1}	Primary or tertiary hyperparathyroidism Malignancy Sarcoidosis Drugs	Confusion Weakness Abdominal pain Hypotension Arrhythmias Cardiac arrest
Hypocalcaemia $[Ca^{2+}]$ <2.1 mmol l^{-1}	Chronic renal failure Acute pancreatitis Calcium channel-blocker overdose Toxic shock syndrome Rhabdomyolysis Tumour lysis syndrome	Paraesthesia Tetany Seizures AV block Cardiac arrest
Hypermagnesaemia $[Mg^{2+}]$ >1.1 mmol l^{-1}	Renal failure Iatrogenic	Confusion Weakness Respiratory depression AV block Cardiac arrest
Hypomagnesaemia $[Mg^{2+}]$ <0.6 mmol l^{-1}	GI loss Polyuria Starvation Alcoholism Malabsorption	Tremor Ataxia Nystagmus Seizures Arrhythmias – torsades de pointes Cardiac arrest

- Airway obstruction and respiratory arrest due to a decreased conscious level is a common cause of death. Alcohol excess is often associated with self-poisoning.
- Avoid mouth-to-mouth resuscitation in the presence of toxins (e.g. cyanide, hydrogen sulphide, corrosives and organophosphates). Use a pocket mask or bag-mask and the highest possible concentration of oxygen for ventilation.

ECG	Treatment
Short QT interval Prolonged QRS Interval Flat T waves AV block Cardiac arrest	Fluid replacement IV Furosemide 1mg kg^{-1} IV Hydrocortisone 200–300 mg IV Pamidronate 60–90 mg IV Calcitonin 4–8 units kg^{-1} 8 h^{-1} IM Review medication Haemodialysis
Prolonged QT interval T-wave inversion Heart block Cardiac arrest	Calcium chloride 10% 10–40 ml Magnesium sulphate 50% 4–8 mmol (if necessary)
Prolonged PR and QT intervals T-wave peaking AV block Cardiac arrest	Calcium chloride 10% 5–10 ml repeated if necessary Ventilatory support if necessary Saline diuresis – 0.9% saline with furosemide 1 mg kg^{-1} IV Haemodialysis
Prolonged PR and QT Intervals ST segment depression T-wave inversion Flattened P waves Increased QRS duration Torsades de pointes	**1. Severe or symptomatic:** 1–2 g 50% magnesium sulphate (2–4 ml; 4–8 mmol) IV over 15 min **2. Torsade de pointes:** 2 g 50% magnesium sulphate (4 ml; 8 mmol) IV over 1–2 min **3. Seizure:** 2 g 50% magnesium sulphate (4 ml; 8 mmol) IV over 10 min

- Pulmonary aspiration of gastric contents common after poisoning. Use a rapid sequence induction with cricoid pressure for tracheal intubation to decrease the risk of aspiration in patients who cannot protect their airway.
- In cardiac arrest provide basic and advanced life support as normal.
- Cardioversion is indicated for life-threatening tachyarrhythmias except torsades de pointes (see peri-arrest arrhythmias).
- Hypotension is common and usually responds to fluid therapy. Occasionally inotropic support is required.
- Once resuscitation is underway, try to identify the poison(s). Relatives, friends and ambulance crews can provide useful information. Patient examination can give clues: odours, needle marks, pinpoint pupils, tablet residues, signs of corrosion in the mouth or blisters associated with prolonged coma.
- Hypo- or hyperthermia can occur after drug overdose.
- Consult regional or national poisons centres for latest specific treatment information.

Specific therapeutic measures

- Emphasis is on intensive supportive therapy, with correction of hypoxia, acid/base and electrolyte disorders.
- Therapeutic measures include limiting absorption of ingested poisons, enhancing elimination or the use of specific antidotes.
- Activated charcoal: consider giving a single dose of activated charcoal to patients who have ingested a potentially toxic amount of poison (known to be adsorbed by activated charcoal) up to 1 h previously. Give only to patients with an intact or protected airway. Multiple doses may be beneficial in life-threatening poisoning with carbemazepine, dapsone, phenobarbital, quinine and theophylline.
- Gastric lavage followed by activated charcoal therapy is useful only within 1 h of ingesting the poison. Ensure airway protection.

- Whole bowel irrigation useful in potentially toxic ingestion of sustained release or enteric coated drugs, oral iron poisoning and the removal of ingested packets of illicit drugs.
- Urine alkalinisation (pH >7.5) by giving IV sodium bicarbonate may be useful in moderate to severe salicylate poisoning in patients who do not need haemodialysis. Urine alkalinisation also useful in tricyclic overdose.
- Haemodialysis useful for poisoning with methanol, ethylene glycol, salicylates and lithium. Charcoal haemoperfusion for intoxications with carbamazepine, phenobarbital, phenytoin and theophylline.
- Specific antidotes include: *N*-acetylcysteine for paracetamol; high-dose atropine for organophosphate insecticides; sodium nitrite, sodium thiosulphate or dicobalt edetate for cyanides; digoxin-specific Fab antibodies for digoxin; flumazenil for benzodiazepines; naloxone for opioids. Reversal of benzodiazepine intoxication with flumazenil is associated with significant toxicity in patients with benzodiazepine dependence or co-ingestion of proconvulsant medications such as tricyclic antidepressants. The routine use of flumazenil in the comatose overdose patient is not recommended.

Specific antidotes

Opioid poisoning

- Respiratory depression is reversed rapidly by naloxone. Use airway opening, oxygen and ventilation before naloxone in patients with opioid-induced respiratory depression.
- Initial doses of naloxone are 0.4 mg IV, 0.8 mg IM, 0.8 mg SC, 2 mg IN and 1–2 mg ET. Large opioid overdoses require titration to a total naloxone dose of 6–10 mg. The clinical effects of naloxone may not last as long as those of a significant opioid overdose.

Titrate the dose until the victim is breathing adequately and has protective airway reflexes.

- Once cardiac arrest has occurred, follow standard resuscitation protocols.

Tricyclic antidepressant poisoning

- Causes hypotension, seizures and arrhythmias. Anticholinergic effects include mydriasis, fever, dry skin, delirium, tachycardia, ileus and urinary retention. Most life-threatening problems occur within the first 6 h after ingestion.
- A widening QRS complex indicates a greater risk of arrhythmias. Consider sodium bicarbonate or hypertonic saline in high-risk patients.

Cocaine toxicity

- Can cause agitation, symptomatic tachycardia, hypertensive crisis, hyperthermia and myocardial ischaemia with angina.
- Glyceryl trinitrate and phentolamine reverse cocaine-induced coronary vasoconstriction. Benzodiazepines (midazolam, diazepam, lorazepam) are effective first-line drugs. Use nitrates only as second-line therapy for myocardial ischaemia. Use labetalol (alpha- and beta-blocker) for treatment of tachycardia and hypertensive emergencies.

Further treatment and prognosis

- Measure electrolytes (particularly potassium), blood glucose and arterial blood gases. Monitor temperature because thermoregulation is impaired. Both hypothermia and hyperthermia (hyperpyrexia) can occur. Retain samples of blood and urine for analysis. Patients may need:
- Higher medication doses than standard protocols.
- Non-standard drug therapies.
- Prolonged CPR.

3. Drowning

Definition

- Drowning is defined as "a process resulting in primary respiratory impairment from submersion/ immersion in a liquid medium. Implicit in this definition is that a liquid/air interface is present at the entrance of the victim's airway, preventing the victim from breathing air. The victim may live or die after this process, but whatever the outcome, he or she has been involved in a drowning incident." Immersion means to be covered in water. Submersion implies that the entire body, including the airway, is under the water or other fluid.

Basic life support

- Ensure personal safety at all times. Whenever possible, try to save the victim without entry into the water. Talking to the victim, reaching with a rescue aid (e.g. stick or clothing) or throwing a rope or buoyant rescue aid may be effective. Alternatively, use a boat or other water vehicle. If entry into the water is essential, take a buoyant rescue aid or flotation device.
- Remove victims from the water by the fastest and safest means available and resuscitate as quickly as possible. Cervical spine immobilisation is not indicated unless signs of severe injury are apparent or the history is consistent with the possibility of severe injury. These circumstances include a history of diving, water slide use, signs of trauma or signs of alcohol intoxication. Despite potential spinal injury, if the victim is pulseless and apnoeic, remove them from the water as quickly as possible (even if a back support device is not available) whilst attempting to limit neck movement. If possible, remove the victim from the water in a horizontal position to minimise the risks of post-immersion hypotension and cardiovascular collapse.

- Early rescue breathing or positive-pressure ventilation increases survival. In the apnoeic victim, start rescue breathing as soon as the victim's airway can be opened and the rescuer's safety ensured. This can sometimes be achieved when the victim is still in shallow water. It is likely to be difficult to pinch the victim's nose, so mouth-to-nose ventilation may be used as an alternative to mouth-to-mouth ventilation. If the victim is in deep water, start in-water rescue breathing if trained to do so; ideally, with the support of a buoyant rescue aid, although in-water unsupported resuscitation may also be possible. Untrained rescuers should not attempt to perform any form of resuscitation with a victim in deep water.
- If there is no spontaneous breathing after opening the airway, give rescue breaths for approximately 1 min. If the victim does not then start breathing spontaneously, further management depends on the distance from land. If the rescuer and victim are close to land (<5 min rescue time) continue rescue breaths whilst towing. If they are more than an estimated 5 min from land, give further rescue breaths over 1 min, and check breathing again. If there are no signs of breathing, bring the victim to land as quickly as possible without further attempts at ventilation. If the victim shows some signs of circulation, continue rescue breathing whilst simultaneously towing to land.
- There is no need to clear the airway of aspirated water. An attempt to remove water from the air passages by any means other than suction is unnecessary and dangerous.
- As soon as the victim is removed from the water, check for breathing. A healthcare professional who is trained in pulse checking may also check for a pulse, but this may be even more difficult to find in a drowning victim, particularly if cold. If the victim is not breathing, start chest compressions immediately. Chest compression is ineffective in the water.

- If there are no signs of life and an AED is available dry the victim's chest and attach it to the victim and activate. Deliver shocks according to the AED prompts. If the patient is hypothermic with a core body temperature ≤30°C (86°F), limit defibrillation to a total of three attempts until the core body temperature rises above 30°C (86°F).
- Regurgitation of stomach contents is common following resuscitation from drowning. If regurgitation occurs, turn the victim's mouth to the side and remove the vomit using directed suction if possible. If spinal cord injury is suspected, remove the vomit by log-rolling the victim, keeping the head, neck and torso aligned. This requires several rescuers.

Advanced life support

- If breathing spontaneously, give high-flow oxygen. Consider non-invasive ventilation or continuous positive airway pressure if severe hypoxia. Use pulse oximetry and arterial blood gas analysis to titrate the concentration of inspired oxygen. Consider early intubation using a rapid sequence induction and controlled ventilation for victims who fail to respond to initial measures or have a reduced level of consciousness.
- Follow standard ALS protocols. If severe hypothermia is present [core body temperature ≤30°C (86°F)], limit defibrillation attempts to three, and withhold intravenous drugs until the core body temperature increases above 30°C. If moderate hypothermia is present, give intravenous drugs at longer than standard intervals.
- During prolonged immersion, victims can become hypovolaemic due to the hydrostatic pressure of the water on the body, inducing a reduction in body fluid volume. Give intravenous fluid to correct hypovolaemia. Avoid excessive volumes, which may cause pulmonary oedema. After ROSC use haemodynamic monitoring to guide fluid resuscitation.

Discontinuing resuscitation efforts

The decision to discontinue resuscitation efforts on a drowning victim is difficult. Continue resuscitation unless there is clear evidence that attempts are futile (e.g. massive traumatic injuries, rigor mortis, putrefaction, etc.), or timely evacuation to a medical facility is not possible. Neurologically intact survival has been reported in several victims submerged for greater than 60 min.

Post-resuscitation care

- There are no clinical differences in the management of salt water or fresh water drowning.
- There is a high risk of acute respiratory distress syndrome (ARDS) for up to 72 h after submersion. Consider protective ventilation strategies using low tidal volumes and positive end expiratory pressure (PEEP).
- Pneumonia is common after drowning. Treatment is based on cultures and microbiology advice.
- If submersion occurs in icy water [<5°C (41°F)], hypothermia develops rapidly and provides some protection against hypoxia. Such effects have typically been reported after submersion of children in *icy* water. Hypothermia may develop as a secondary complication of the submersion, and subsequent heat loss through evaporation, during attempted resuscitation. In these victims the hypothermia is not protective.
- Consider instituting active re-warming until a core temperature of 32–34°C is achieved and then actively to avoid hyperthermia (>37°C) during the subsequent period of intensive care (International Life Saving Federation, 2003).

4. Hypothermia

Definition

- Hypothermia exists when the body core temperature is below 35°C.

- Classified arbitrarily as mild (35–32°C), moderate (32–30°C) or severe (<30°C).
- Occurs in people with normal thermoregulation who are exposed to cold environments, particularly wet or windy conditions, or following immersion in cold water. With impaired thermoregulation (e.g. in the elderly and very young) hypothermia may follow a mild cold insult. Risk increased by drug or alcohol ingestion, illness, injury or neglect.
- Hypothermia may be suspected from the clinical history or a brief external examination of a collapsed patient. A low reading thermometer is needed to measure the core temperature and confirm the diagnosis.

Decision to resuscitate

- Beware of pronouncing death in a hypothermic patient, as cold alone may produce a very slow, small volume, irregular pulse and an unrecordable blood pressure.
- Dilated pupils can be caused by a variety of insults and must not be taken as a sign of death.
- Cardiac arrest could be due primarily to hypothermia, or secondary to a normothermic cardiac arrest (e.g. cardiac arrest due to myocardial ischaemia in a person in a cold environment).
- Do not confirm death until the patient has been re-warmed, or attempts to raise the core temperature have failed; prolonged resuscitation may be necessary. In the pre-hospital setting, withhold resuscitation if the patient has obvious lethal injuries or if the body is completely frozen, making resuscitation attempts impossible. In the hospital setting, use clinical judgement to determine when to stop resuscitation.

Resuscitation

All the principles of prevention, basic and advanced life support apply to the hypothermic patient.

- Clear the airway and, if there is no spontaneous respiratory effort, ventilate the patient's lungs with high concentrations of oxygen. Use warmed (40–46°C) and humidified oxygen. Consider careful tracheal intubation (may provoke VF) if indicated according to the ALS algorithm.
- Palpate a major artery, look for signs of life and, if available, look at the ECG for up to 1 min before concluding that there is no cardiac output. If a Doppler ultrasound probe is available use it to establish if there is peripheral blood flow. If the victim is pulseless with no detectable signs of circulation, start chest compressions immediately. If there is any doubt about whether a pulse is present, start CPR.
- Confirm hypothermia with a low reading thermometer.
- Use the same ventilation and chest compression rates as for a normothermic patient.
- Withhold adrenaline and other drugs until the patient has been warmed to a temperature greater than 30°C. Once 30°C has been reached, the intervals between doses should be doubled. As the patient's temperature returns towards normal the standard drug protocols should be used.
- Rule out other primary causes of cardiac arrest using the four Hs and four Ts approach.
- As temperature decreases, sinus bradycardia tends to give way to atrial fibrillation followed by ventricular fibrillation (VF) and, finally, asystole. Follow standard treatment protocols.
- Arrhythmias other than VF tend to revert spontaneously as the core temperature increases and usually do not require immediate treatment. Bradycardia may be physiological in severe hypothermia, and cardiac pacing is not indicated unless the bradycardia persists after re-warming.
- If VF is detected, give a shock; if VF/VT persists after three shocks, delay further defibrillation attempts until

the core temperature is above 30°C. If an AED is used, follow the AED prompts whilst re-warming the patient.

Re-warming

- General measures include removal from the cold, preventing further heat loss and rapid transfer to hospital. Remove cold or wet clothing as soon as practical. Dry the casualty, cover with blankets and keep them out of the wind.
- Re-warming can be passive external, active external or active internal. Passive warming is achieved with blankets and a warm room and is suitable for conscious victims with mild hypothermia. Forced air re-warming and warm IV fluids are effective in patients with severe hypothermia and a perfusing rhythm.
- Consider warm humidified gases and gastric, peritoneal, pleural or bladder lavage with warm fluids (at 40°C), and extracorporeal blood warming with partial bypass.
- In cardiac arrest and hypothermia, cardiopulmonary bypass is the preferred method of active internal re-warming because it also provides circulation, oxygenation and ventilation while the core body temperature is increased gradually.
- Once ROSC has been achieved, use standard strategies for post-resuscitation care, including mild hypothermia if appropriate.

5. Hyperthermia

- Hyperthermia occurs along a continuum of heat-related conditions starting with heat stress, progressing to heat exhaustion, heat stroke (HS) and culminating in multi-organ dysfunction and cardiac arrest in some instances.
- Malignant hyperthermia (MH) is a rare disorder characterised by muscle contracture and hypermetabolic crisis following exposure of

genetically predisposed individuals to halogenated anaesthetics and depolarising muscle relaxants.

The key features and treatment of heat stress and heat exhaustion are included in Table 6.2.

Table 6.2 Heat stress and heat exhaustion

	Features	Treatment
Heat stress	Normal or mild temperature elevation Heat oedema – swelling of feet and ankles Heat syncope – vasodilation causing hypotension Heat cramps – sodium depletion causing cramps	Rest Elevation of oedematous limbs Cooling Oral rehydration Salt replacement
Heat exhaustion	Systemic reaction to prolonged heat exposure (hours to days) Temperature >37°C and <40°C Headache, dizziness, nausea, vomiting Tachycardia, hypotension Sweating Muscle pain, weakness and cramps Haemoconcentration Hyponatraemia or hypernatraemia May progress rapidly to heat stroke	As above Consider IV fluids and ice packs for severe cases

Heat stroke

- Systemic inflammatory response with a core temperature above 40.6°C accompanied by mental state change and varying levels of organ dysfunction. Mortality between 10% and 50%.
- Classic non-exertional heat stroke (CHS) occurs during high environmental temperatures and often affects the elderly during heat waves.

- Exertional heat stroke (EHS) occurs during strenuous physical exercise in high environmental temperatures and/or high humidity. Usually affects healthy young adults.
- Elderly are at increased risk for heat-related illness because of underlying illness, medication use, declining thermoregulatory mechanisms and limited social support.
- Risk factors include: lack of acclimatisation, dehydration, obesity, alcohol, cardiovascular disease, skin conditions (psoriasis, eczema, scleroderma, burn, cystic fibrosis), hyperthyroidism, phaeochromocytoma and drugs (anticholinergics, heroin, cocaine, amphetamine, phenothiazines, sympathomimetics, calcium channel-blockers, beta-blockers).

Recognition

- Heat stroke can resemble septic shock. Features include: core temperature 40.6°C or more; hot, dry skin (sweating is present in half of the cases of exertional heat stroke); extreme fatigue, headache, fainting, facial flushing, vomiting and diarrhoea; cardiovascular dysfunction including arrhythmias and hypotension; respiratory dysfunction including ARDS; central nervous system dysfunction including seizures and coma; liver and renal failure; coagulopathy; and rhabdomyolysis.
- Other clinical conditions need to be considered, including: drug toxicity, drug withdrawal syndrome, serotonin syndrome, neuroleptic malignant syndrome, sepsis, central nervous system infection and endocrine disorders, e.g. thyroid storm, phaeochromocytoma.

Management

- Supportive therapy based on optimising the ABCDEs and cooling the patient.
- Start cooling before the patient reaches hospital. Aim to reduce the core temperature to approximately 39°C.

- Use haemodynamic monitoring to guide fluid therapy. Large volumes of fluid may be required. Correct electrolyte abnormalities.
- Simple cooling techniques include drinking cool fluids, fanning the completely undressed patient and spraying tepid water on the patient. Ice packs over areas where there are large superficial blood vessels (axillae, groins, neck) may also be useful.
- Surface cooling methods may cause shivering. In cooperative stable patients, immersion in cold water can be effective. This can cause peripheral vasoconstriction, shunt blood away from the periphery and reduce heat dissipation. Immersion is not practical in the sickest patients.
- Gastric, peritoneal, pleural or bladder lavage with cold water will lower the core temperature. Intravascular cooling techniques include the use of cold IV fluids, intravascular cooling catheters and extracorporeal circuits, e.g. continuous veno–veno haemofiltration or cardiopulmonary bypass.

Malignant hyperthermia

- Life-threatening genetic sensitivity of skeletal muscles to volatile anaesthetics and depolarising neuromuscular-blocking drugs occurring during or after anaesthesia. Stop triggering agents immediately; give oxygen, correct acidosis and electrolyte abnormalities. Start active cooling and give dantrolene.

Modifications to cardiopulmonary resuscitation and post-resuscitation care

- Follow standard protocols for basic and advanced life support and cool the patient. Provide post-resuscitation care according to normal guidelines.

6. Asthma

Causes of cardiac arrest

- Cardiac arrest in the asthmatic is often a terminal event after a period of hypoxaemia. Cardiac arrest in asthmatics has been linked to: severe bronchospasm and mucous plugging leading to asphyxia, cardiac arrhythmias due to hypoxia, dynamic hyperinflation [auto-positive end expiratory pressure (auto-PEEP) can occur in mechanically ventilated asthmatics] and tension pneumothorax (often bilateral).

- Use the four Hs and four Ts approach to identify reversible causes of cardiac arrest.

Recognition

The severity of an asthma attack is defined in Table 6.3.

Interventions to prevent arrest in near-fatal asthma

- The patient with severe asthma requires aggressive medical management.
- Base assessment and treatment on an ABCDE approach. Experienced clinicians should treat these high-risk patients in a critical care area. Specific drugs and the treatment sequence will vary according to local practice.
- Give inspired oxygen to achieve an oxygen saturation (SaO_2) of ≥92%. High-flow oxygen by mask is sometimes necessary.
- Consider rapid sequence induction and tracheal intubation if, despite efforts to optimise drug therapy, the patient has: decreasing conscious level, coma; profuse sweating; poor ('floppy') muscle tone (clinical signs of hypercarbia); findings of severe agitation, confusion and fighting against the oxygen mask (clinical signs of hypoxaemia); elevation of the $PaCO_2$ alone does not indicate the need for tracheal intubation. Treat the patient, not the numbers.
- Give salbutamol (5 mg nebulised). Repeated doses every 15–20 min or continuous nebulised salbutamol may be needed. Use nebuliser units that can be driven by high-flow oxygen. Hypoventilation associated with severe or near-fatal asthma may prevent effective delivery of nebulised drugs.

Table 6.3 The severity of asthma

Table 6.3 The severity of asthma
Near-fatal asthma
Raised $PaCO_2$ and/or requiring mechanical ventilation with raised inflation pressures
Life-threatening asthma
Any one of the following in a patient with severe asthma: • Peak expiratory flow (PEF) <33% best or predicted • Bradycardia • SpO_2 <92% • Dysrhythmia • PaO_2 <8 kPa • Hypotension • Normal $PaCO_2$ (4.6–6.0 kPa) • Exhaustion • Silent chest • Confusion • Cyanosis • Coma • Feeble respiratory effort
Acute severe asthma
Any one of: • PEF 33–50% best or predicted • Respiratory rate >25 min^{-1} • Heart rate >110 min^{-1} • Inability to complete sentences in one breath
Moderate asthma exacerbation
• Increasing symptoms • PEF >50–75% best or predicted • No features of acute severe asthma
Brittle asthma
• Type 1: wide PEF variability (>40% diurnal variation for >50% of the time over a period >150 d) despite intense therapy • Type 2: sudden severe attacks on a background of apparently well controlled asthma

- Give corticosteroids (hydrocortisone 200 mg IV) early.
- Nebulised anticholinergics (ipratropium 0.5 mg 4–6 hourly) may produce additional bronchodilation in severe asthma.
- Intravenous salbutamol (250 mcg IV slowly) to provide additional benefit in severe asthmatics who are

already receiving nebulised salbutamol. An infusion of 3–20 mcg min^{-1} may be given.

- Magnesium sulphate (2 g IV slowly) may be useful as a bronchodilator in severe or near-fatal asthma.
- Aminophylline should only be considered in severe or near-fatal asthma. A loading dose of 5 mg kg^{-1} is given over 20–30 min (unless on maintenance therapy) followed by an infusion of 0.5–0.7 mg kg^{-1} h^{-1}. Addition to high doses of β_2-agonists increases side-effects more than it increases bronchodilation. Check levels to avoid toxicity.
- If there is evidence of hypovolaemia or dehydration, give intravenous fluids.
- Other therapies such as non-invasive ventilation, helium oxygen mixtures and ketamine can be considered by those expert in their use.

Management of cardiac arrest

Basic life support

Follow standard guidelines. Ventilation will be difficult because of increased airway resistance; try to prevent gastric inflation.

Advanced life support

- Intubate the trachea early to make ventilation easier and prevent gastric insufflation.
- The recommended respiratory rate (10 breaths min^{-1}) and tidal volume required for a normal chest rise during CPR should not cause dynamic hyperinflation of the lungs (gas trapping).
- If dynamic hyperinflation of the lungs is suspected during CPR, compression of the chest wall and/or a period of apnoea (disconnection of tracheal tube) may relieve gas trapping if dynamic hyperinflation occurs.
- Dynamic hyperinflation increases transthoracic impedance. Consider higher shock energies for defibrillation if initial defibrillation attempts fail.

Post-resuscitation care

- Optimise the medical management of bronchospasm.
- It may not be possible to achieve normal oxygenation and ventilation in a patient with severe bronchospasm. Efforts to achieve normal arterial blood gas values may worsen lung injury. Mild hypoventilation reduces the risk of barotrauma and hypercapnia is typically well tolerated. Target lower arterial blood oxygen saturations (e.g. 90%).
- Provide sedation (neuromuscular paralysis if needed) and controlled ventilation. Ketamine and inhalational anaesthetics have bronchodilator properties that may be useful in asthmatic patients who are difficult to ventilate.

7. Anaphylaxis

- Anaphylaxis is a hypersensitivity reaction mediated typically by immunoglobulin E (IgE).
- Anaphylactoid reactions are similar, but do not depend upon hypersensitivity.
- The treatment is the same. Anaphylaxis will be used to describe both types of reaction.
- Anaphylactic reaction is a severe, systemic allergic reaction with multisystem involvement, involving the airway, vascular system, gastrointestinal tract and skin. Severe cases may cause complete airway obstruction secondary to laryngeal oedema, bronchospasm, hypotension, cardiovascular collapse and death. Other symptoms include rhinitis, conjunctivitis, abdominal pain, vomiting, diarrhoea and a sense of impending doom. The patient may appear either flushed or pale.
- Anaphylactic reactions vary in severity. Progress may be rapid, slow or (unusually) biphasic. Rarely, manifestations may be delayed (this may occur with latex allergy), or persist for more than 24 h.
- Anaphylaxis is caused by a hypersensitivity reaction in which histamine, serotonin and other vasoactive

substances are released from basophils and mast cells in response to an IgE-mediated reaction. Antigen-specific immunoglobulins are produced after initial exposure to an allergen. Subsequent re-exposure to this allergen provokes an anaphylactic reaction, although many anaphylactic reactions occur without known prior exposure.

- Although anaphylaxis is relatively common, progression to a severe life-threatening reaction is rare. Any antigen capable of activating IgE can theoretically be a trigger for anaphylaxis. The commonest causes of life-threatening reactions are drugs, stinging insects and food. In as many as 5% of cases the antigen triggering the anaphylaxis cannot be identified.
- Neuromuscular-blocking drugs and antibiotics are the commonest triggers for drug-induced anaphylaxis.
- Latex, or natural rubber, is a common trigger among hospitalised patients because of frequent instrumentation and operations in which latex products are used. Avoidance of latex is the only effective therapy. Deaths from latex allergy are rare.
- The prevalence of IgE-mediated systemic reactions is more common in countries such as Australia where exposure to insect stings is more common. The stinging insects include hornets, wasps, honey bees and fire ants. Most stings cause local reactions with pain and swelling at the site, but progress to anaphylaxis in susceptible persons. Fatal anaphylaxis occurs in people who are re-stung after a prior sting has induced IgE antibodies. Fatal reactions occur within 10–15 min, with cardiovascular collapse being the commonest cause of death.
- Peanuts, seafood (in particular prawns and shellfish) and wheat are the most frequent foods associated with life-threatening anaphylaxis. Bronchospasm, angioedema, airway obstruction and asphyxia comprise the most frequent fatal mechanism.

Signs and symptoms

- Considered when two or more body systems are affected (cutaneous, respiratory, cardiovascular, neurological or gastrointestinal), with or without cardiovascular or airway involvement. Symptoms may be severe in patients with asthma, those taking beta-adrenoceptor blockers and during neuraxial anaesthesia, states associated with reduced endogenous catecholamine response. The speed of onset of signs and symptoms is related to the likely severity of the ensuing anaphylaxis.
- Signs and symptoms include: urticaria, rhinitis, conjunctivitis, abdominal pain, vomiting and diarrhoea. Flushing is common, but pallor may also occur. Marked upper airway (laryngeal) oedema and bronchospasm may develop, causing stridor and wheezing (or high airway pressures in ventilated patients). Cardiovascular collapse is the most common peri-arrest manifestation. Vasodilation causes relative hypovolaemia, exacerbated by true volume loss as increased capillary permeability results in extravasation of intravascular fluid. Additional cardiac dysfunction may follow from underlying disease or from the development of myocardial ischaemia from adrenaline administration.
- The wide range of possible presentations may cause diagnostic difficulty. The history of previous allergic reactions is important as well as that of the recent incident. Pay particular attention to the condition of the skin, the pulse rate, the blood pressure and the upper airways, and auscultate the chest. Measure and record peak flow where possible. Consider the diagnosis of other conditions only after anaphylaxis has been excluded; failure to identify and treat anaphylaxis can be fatal.
- ACE inhibitors may cause angioedema with marked swelling of the upper airway. This reaction may occur at any time and is not related to initial exposure to the

drug. The best treatment for this form of angioedema is unclear, but early recognition and appropriate airway management is critical.

- Hereditary angioedema is familial and indistinguishable from the early angioedema of anaphylaxis or drug-related angioedema. An important distinguishing feature is the absence of urticaria with hereditary angioedema. This is treated with C1 esterase inhibitor, either as a specific concentrate or contained within fresh frozen plasma.
- Severe asthma may present with bronchospasm and stridor, which are also common features of severe anaphylaxis. However, asthma attacks do not usually present with urticaria or angioedema.
- Rarely, panic attacks may be associated with functional stridor as a result of forced adduction of the vocal cords. As with asthma, there is no urticaria, angioedema, hypoxia or hypotension.
- Vasovagal reactions cause sudden collapse and extreme bradycardia that may be mistaken for absence of a pulse. Recovery is usually relatively rapid and is not associated with urticaria, angioedema or bronchospasm.

General resuscitation measures

- Victims should recline in a position of comfort. Remove the likely allergen (i.e. stop drug infusion or blood transfusion). Lying flat with or without leg elevation may be helpful for hypotension but unhelpful for breathing difficulties.
- Airway obstruction can develop rapidly due to soft tissue swelling. Consider early tracheal intubation; delay may make intubation extremely difficult.
- Give high-flow oxygen (10–15 litres min^{-1}).
- Give adrenaline intramuscularly to all patients with clinical signs of shock, airway swelling or definite breathing difficulty; it will be absorbed rapidly. Inspiratory stridor, wheeze, cyanosis, pronounced tachycardia and decreased capillary filling indicate

a severe reaction. For adults, give an intramuscular dose of 0.5 ml adrenaline 1:1000 solution (500 μg). If the patient's condition fails to improve, repeat the dose after about 5 min. In some cases several doses may be needed, particularly if improvement is transient.

- Doctors experienced in the use of intravenous adrenaline may prefer to use the intravenous route in any patient with signs of severe anaphylaxis. Intravenous adrenaline (in a dilution of at least 1:10,000) is hazardous and must be reserved for patients with profound shock that is immediately life-threatening and for special indications, for example during anaesthesia. This should be carried out with a minimum of electrocardiographic monitoring.
- Give an H_1-antihistamine (e.g. chlorphenamine 10–20 mg) by slow IV injection. Consider also an H_2-blocker, e.g. ranitidine (50 mg IV).
- Give hydrocortisone by slow intravenous injection after severe attacks to help avert late sequelae. Corticosteroids are considered as slow-acting drugs but may help in the emergency treatment of an acute attack. They also have a role in preventing or shortening protracted reactions.
- An inhaled β_2-agonist such as salbutamol (5 mg repeated if necessary) may help reverse refractory bronchospasm. Consider inhaled ipratropium (500 μg, repeated as necessary).
- If severe hypotension does not respond rapidly to drug treatment, give fluid; a rapid infusion of 1–2 litres may be required. Further fluid is likely to be required.
- There is some evidence for vasopressin in severe hypotension; glucagon for those on beta-blockers.
- Rarely, insect envenomation by bees, but not wasps, leaves a venom sac. Immediately scrape away any insect parts at the site of the sting. Squeezing may increase envenomation.

Cardiac arrest

- Follow standard BLS and ALS protocols.
- Near-fatal anaphylaxis produces profound vasodilation and a relative hypovolaemia. Massive volume replacement is essential. Use at least two large-bore cannulae with pressure bags to give large volumes (as much as 4–8 litres of intravenous fluid may be necessary in the immediate resuscitation period).
- Give an antihistamine intravenously if one has not already been given before the arrest.
- Steroids given during a cardiac arrest will have little immediate effect, but if ROSC is restored, they may be effective in the post-resuscitation period.
- Patients with anaphylaxis are often young, with healthy hearts and cardiovascular systems. Effective CPR may maintain sufficient oxygen delivery until the catastrophic effects of the anaphylactic reaction resolve, i.e. prolonged CPR may be necessary.

Airway obstruction

Airway obstruction may occur rapidly in severe anaphylaxis, particularly in patients with angioedema. Warning signs are lingual and labial swelling, hoarseness and oropharyngeal swelling. Consider early, elective intubation. As airway obstruction progresses, both LMA and Combitube are likely to be difficult to insert. Tracheal intubation and cricothyroidotomy will also become increasingly difficult. Attempts at tracheal intubation may exacerbate laryngeal oedema. Early involvement of a senior anaesthetist is mandatory when managing these patients.

Observation

Warn patients with even moderate attacks of the possibility of an early recurrence of symptoms and in some circumstances keep them under observation for 8–24 h. This caution is particularly applicable to: severe reactions with slow onset due to idiopathic anaphylaxis; reactions in severe asthmatics or with a severe asthmatic component; reactions with the possibility of continuing absorption of allergen; patients with a previous history of biphasic reactions.

Investigations and further management

Measurement of mast cell tryptase may help with retrospective diagnosis of anaphylaxis. Take three 10 ml clotted blood samples: 1) immediately after the reaction has been treated; 2) about 1 h after the reaction; 3) about 6 h and up to 24 h after the reaction.

Refer the patient to a specialist clinic. Patients at very high risk of anaphylaxis may carry their own adrenaline syringe for self-administration and wear a 'medic-alert' type bracelet. Report any adverse drug reactions.

8. Traumatic cardiorespiratory arrest (TCRA)

- Cardiac arrest secondary to traumatic injury has a very low survival (2.2%).
- The diagnosis of TCRA is made clinically: the trauma patient is unresponsive, apnoeic and pulseless. Both asystole and organised cardiac activity without cardiac output are regarded as TCRA.
- Commotio cordis is actual or near cardiac arrest caused by a blunt impact to the chest wall over the heart (usually during sport). A blow to the chest during the vulnerable phase of the cardiac cycle may cause malignant arrhythmias (usually ventricular fibrillation).
- Cardiac arrest due to a medical pathology (e.g. cardiac arrhythmia, hypoglycaemia, seizure) may cause a secondary traumatic event (e.g. fall, road traffic accident, etc.).

Signs of life and initial ECG activity

- There are no reliable predictors of survival for TCRA.
- The American College of Surgeons and the National Association of EMS physicians produced pre-hospital guidelines that recommend withholding resuscitation in:

1. Blunt trauma patients presenting with apnoea, pulselessness and without organised ECG activity.
2. Penetrating trauma patients found apnoeic and pulseless after rapid assessment for signs of life such as pupillary reflexes, spontaneous movement or organised ECG activity.

Treatment

- Prolonged CPR is associated with a poor outcome.
- Treatment on scene should focus on good quality BLS and ALS and exclusion of reversible causes.
- Look for and treat any medical condition that may have precipitated the trauma event.
- Undertake only essential life-saving interventions on scene and, if the patient has signs of life, transfer rapidly to the nearest appropriate hospital.
- Consider on-scene thoracotomy for appropriate patients.
- Do not delay for unproven interventions such as spinal immobilisation.

Resuscitative thoracotomy

Pre-hospital: one UK service recommends that if surgical intervention cannot be accomplished within 10 min after loss of pulse in patients with penetrating chest injury, on-scene thoracotomy should be considered.

Hospital: the American College of Surgeons has published practice guidelines for emergency department thoracotomy (EDT).These state that:

1. After blunt trauma, EDT should be limited to those with vital signs on arrival and a witnessed cardiac arrest (estimated survival rate 1.6%).
2. Emergency department thoracotomy is best applied to patients with penetrating cardiac injuries who arrive at the trauma centre after a short on-scene and transport time with witnessed signs of life or ECG activity (estimated survival rate 31%).
3. Emergency department thoracotomy should be undertaken in penetrating non-cardiac thoracic injuries even though survival rates are low.

4. Emergency department thoracotomy should be undertaken in patients with exsanguinating abdominal vascular injury even though survival rates are low. This procedure should be used as an adjunct to definitive repair of abdominal vascular injury.

Airway and breathing management

- Tracheal intubation on scene of patients with TCRA may double the tolerated period of CPR.
- Use basic airway management manoeuvres and alternative airways to maintain oxygenation if tracheal intubation cannot be accomplished immediately. If these measures fail a surgical airway is indicated.
- Monitor ventilation with capnometry and adjust to achieve normocapnia.
- Excessive ventilation and increased intrathoracic pressure lowers cardiac output.
- Decompression of a tension pneumothorax can be achieved quickly by lateral thoracostomy. This is more effective than needle thoracostomy and quicker than inserting a chest tube.

Circulation management

- In hypovolaemic cardiac arrest or cardiac tamponade, chest compressions are less effective as in cardiac arrest from other causes.
- Chest compressions are still the standard of care in patients with cardiac arrest irrespective of aetiology.
- Early haemorrhage control is vital. Handle the patient gently at all times to prevent clot disruption. Apply external compression, and pelvic and limb splints when appropriate. Delays in surgical haemostasis are disastrous for patients with exsanguinating trauma.
- In trauma-related cardiac tamponade, needle pericardiocentesis is probably not a useful procedure. It may increase scene time, can cause myocardial injury and delays effective therapeutic measures such as emergency thoracotomy.

- General consensus supports a conservative approach to intravenous fluid infusion, with permissive hypotension until surgical haemostasis is achieved.
- Some recommend giving 250 ml boluses of crystalloid solution until a radial pulse is achieved and not delaying rapid transport of trauma victims for fluid infusion in the field. Pre-hospital fluid therapy may have a role in prolonged entrapments.
- Ultrasound is a valuable tool in the evaluation of the compromised trauma patient. Haemoperitoneum, haemo- or pneumothorax and cardiac tamponade can be diagnosed reliably in minutes even in the pre-hospital phase.

9. Cardiac arrest associated with pregnancy

- Physiological changes occur during pregnancy – for example, cardiac output, blood volume, minute ventilation and oxygen consumption all increase. Furthermore, the gravid uterus may cause significant compression of iliac and abdominal vessels when the mother is in the supine position, resulting in reduced cardiac output and hypotension.
- Units likely to deal with cardiac arrest in pregnancy should: have plans and equipment for both resuscitation of the pregnant and newborn in place; ensure early involvement of obstetric and neonatal teams; ensure regular training in obstetric emergencies.

Causes

- There are many causes of cardiac arrest in pregnant women. Common causes include: pre-existing cardiac disease, thromboembolism, suicide, hypertensive disorders of pregnancy, sepsis, ectopic pregnancy, haemorrhage, amniotic fluid embolism.
- Pregnant women can also suffer the same causes of cardiac arrest as females of the same age group.

Key interventions to prevent arrest

Use an ABCDE approach. To treat a distressed or compromised pregnant patient:

- Place the patient in the left lateral position or **manually and gently** displace the uterus to the left.
- Give 100% oxygen.
- Give a fluid bolus.
- Immediately re-evaluate the need for any drugs being given.
- Seek expert help early.

Modifications to BLS and ALS guidelines for arrest

- After 20 weeks gestation the pregnant woman's uterus can press down against the inferior vena cava and the aorta, impeding venous return and cardiac output. Upon cardiac arrest, the compromise in venous return and cardiac output by the gravid uterus limits the effectiveness of chest compressions.
- The gravid uterus is shifted away from the cava in most cases by placing the patient in 15 degrees of left lateral decubitus position. Tilt may be accomplished by manual or mechanical means.
- A hand position higher than the centre of the chest may be needed to adjust for the elevation of the diaphragm and abdominal contents caused by the gravid uterus.
- Attempt defibrillation using standard energy doses. Left lateral tilt and large breasts will make it difficult to place an apical defibrillator paddle. Adhesive defibrillator pads are preferable to paddles in pregnancy.
- Early tracheal intubation with correctly applied cricoid pressure decreases this risk of gastric aspiration of gastric contents. It will also make ventilation of the lungs easier in the presence of increased intra-abdominal pressure.
- Tracheal intubation is more difficult in the pregnant patient. Expert help, a failed intubation drill and the use of alternative airway devices may be needed.

Reversible causes

- The 4Hs and 4Ts approach helps identify all the common causes of cardiac arrest in pregnancy.
- Abdominal ultrasound by a skilled operator to detect pregnancy and possible causes during cardiac arrest in pregnancy; however, do not delay other treatments.
- Haemorrhage can occur both antenatally and postnatally. Associations include ectopic pregnancy, placental abruption, placenta praevia and uterine rupture. Treatment is based on an ABCDE approach. The key step is to stop the bleeding. Consider the following: fluid resuscitation including use of rapid transfusion system and cell salvage; correction of coagulopathy; oxytocin and prostaglandins to correct uterine atony; uterine compression sutures; radiological embolisation; hysterectomy; and aortic cross-clamping in catastrophic haemorrhage.
- Iatrogenic overdose is possible in eclamptic women receiving magnesium sulphate, particularly if the woman becomes oliguric. Give calcium to treat magnesium toxicity (see life-threatening electrolyte abnormalities).
- Central neural blockade for analgesia or anaesthesia may cause problems due to sympathetic blockade (hypotension, bradycardia) or local anaesthetic toxicity.
- Pulmonary hypertension causes most deaths from congenital heart disease. Peri-partum cardiomyopathy, myocardial infarction, aneurysm or dissection of the aorta or its branches cause most deaths from acquired cardiac disease. Patients with known cardiac disease need to be managed in a specialist unit.
- Eclampsia is the development of convulsions and/or unexplained coma during pregnancy or post-partum in patients with signs and symptoms of pre-eclampsia. Magnesium sulphate prevents half of the cases of eclampsia developing in women with pre-eclampsia.
- Fibrinolytics for massive pulmonary embolism in pregnant women have been reported.

- Amniotic fluid embolism may present with breathlessness, cyanosis, arrhythmias, hypotension and haemorrhage associated with disseminated intravascular coagulopathy. Treatment is supportive as there is no specific therapy.

If immediate resuscitation attempts fail

- When initial resuscitation attempts fail, delivery of the fetus may improve the chances of successful resuscitation of the mother and fetus. The best survival rate for infants over 24–25 weeks gestation occurs when delivery of the infant is achieved within 5 min after the mother's cardiac arrest.
- This requires that the provider commence the hysterotomy at about 4 min after cardiac arrest.
- Delivery relieves caval compression and enables newborn resuscitation.

Decision making

- **Gestational age <20 weeks**: urgent Caesarean delivery need not be considered, because a gravid uterus of this size is unlikely to significantly compromise maternal cardiac output.
- **Gestational age approximately 20–23 weeks**: initiate emergency hysterotomy to enable successful resuscitation of the mother, not survival of the delivered infant, which is unlikely at this gestational age.
- **Gestational age approximately ≥24–25 weeks**: initiate emergency hysterotomy to save the life of both the mother and the infant.

10. Electrocution

Introduction

- Factors influencing the severity of electrical injury include whether the current is alternating (AC) or direct (DC), voltage, magnitude of energy delivered, resistance to current flow, pathway of current through the patient, and the area and duration of contact. Skin resistance is decreased by moisture, which increases the likelihood of injury.

- Electric current follows the path of least resistance; conductive neurovascular bundles within limbs are particularly prone to damage.
- Contact with AC may cause tetanic contraction of skeletal muscle, which may prevent release from the source of electricity. Myocardial or respiratory failure may cause immediate death:
- *Respiratory arrest* may be caused by paralysis of the central respiratory control system or the respiratory muscles.
- Current may precipitate *ventricular fibrillation* (VF) if it traverses the myocardium during the vulnerable period (analogous to an R-on-T phenomenon). Electrical current may also cause myocardial ischaemia because of coronary artery spasm. *Asystole* may be primary, or secondary to asphyxia following respiratory arrest.

Lightning strike

- Lightning strikes deliver as much as 300 kilovolts over a few milliseconds.
- Most current from a lightning strike passes over the surface of the body.
- Both industrial shocks and lightning strikes cause deep burns at the contact point.
- Injury may also occur through ground current or current 'splashing' from other objects hit by lightning. Explosive force may cause blunt trauma.
- In those who survive the initial shock, extensive catecholamine release or autonomic stimulation may occur, causing hypertension, tachycardia, non-specific ECG changes (including prolongation of the QT interval and transient T-wave inversion) and myocardial necrosis.
- Creatine kinase may be released from myocardial and skeletal muscle.

- Lightning can cause central and peripheral nerve damage.
- Mortality is as high as 30% with up to 70% of survivors sustaining significant morbidity.

Rescue

- Ensure that the power source is switched off. Do not approach the casualty until it is safe.
- High voltage (above domestic mains) electricity can 'arc' and conduct through the ground for up to a few metres around the casualty.

Resuscitation

- Electrical burns around the face and neck can cause soft tissue oedema and airway obstruction. Consider early tracheal intubation and cervical spine control.
- Muscular paralysis can persist for several hours. Ventilatory support will be needed.
- Ventricular fibrillation is the commonest initial arrhythmia after high voltage AC shock. Asystole is more common after DC shock. Use standard BLS and ALS protocols.
- Remove smouldering clothing and shoes to prevent further thermal injury.
- Vigorous fluid therapy is required if there is significant tissue destruction. Maintain a good urine output to enhance the excretion of products of tissue damage.
- Consider early surgical intervention in patients with severe thermal injuries.
- Maintain spinal immobilisation if there is likelihood of head or neck trauma.
- Do a secondary survey to exclude traumatic injuries.
- Electrocution can cause severe, deep soft tissue injury with relatively minor skin wounds; look carefully for features of compartment syndrome, which will necessitate fasciotomy.

11. Cardiac arrest following cardiac surgery

- Cardiac arrest following major cardiac surgery (both on and off bypass) is relatively common in the immediate post-operative phase, with a reported incidence of 0.7% in the first 24 h and 1.4% within the first 8 d.
- Survival to hospital discharge of patients suffering cardiac arrest during the first 24 h after adult cardiac surgery is reported as 54–79% and 41% in children.

Aetiology

- Peri-operative myocardial infarction is often secondary to graft occlusion.
- The main causes of cardiac arrest in the initial post-operative period are: myocardial ischaemia; tension pneumothorax; haemorrhage causing hypovolaemic shock; cardiac tamponade; disconnection of pacing system in pacing-dependent patient; electrolyte disturbances (particularly hypo/hyperkalaemia).

Diagnosis

- Auscultation of the chest, examination of the ECG and chest radiograph, transoesophageal/transthoracic echocardiography and measurement of blood loss from chest drains will aid in identifying the cause of the arrest.
- Exclude reversible causes of cardiac arrest: the four Hs and four Ts.
- Lack of drainage of blood from the chest drains does not exclude haemorrhage or tamponade because drains may block with clot.

Treatment

- Follow standard BLS and ALS protocols.
- Seek assistance from senior clinicians without delay.
- Exclude immediately correctable causes such as pacing lead disconnection and tension pneumothorax.

Extreme bradycardia or asystole may respond to pacing via internal pacing wires (if present) connected to an external pacemaker.

- Be careful when giving intravenous adrenaline as the resulting hypertension may cause catastrophic failure of anastomoses.

Chest compressions

- External chest compressions can cause sternal subluxation, fractured ribs and damage to grafts. Continuous observation of the invasive blood pressure will enable the force of compression to be optimised. Effective external chest compressions should take precedence over concerns of damage to grafts.
- Up to 10% of patients may need chest reopening following cardiac surgery as mechanical factors (e.g. haemorrhage, tamponade, graft occlusion) can cause sudden cardiac arrest in haemodynamically stable patients post-operatively.
- Cardiac arrest on the ICU, arrest within 24 h of surgery and reopening within 10 min of arrest are independent predictors of survival.
- Reopen the patient's chest immediately if there is no output with external cardiac massage or if there is a shockable rhythm refractory to cardioversion. Management of asystole usually requires prompt chest opening.
- Consider training non-surgical medical staff to open the wound and remove sternal wires while a surgeon is summoned.
- Early identification and treatment of underlying pathology is challenging under theses circumstances and requires an experienced surgeon.

Re-institution of emergency cardiopulmonary bypass

- Emergency institution of CPB should be available on all units undertaking cardiac surgery. Survival to discharge rates of up to 56.3% have been reported when CPB is re-instituted on the ICU.

- Ensuring adequate re-anticoagulation prior to commencing CPB or the use of a heparin-bonded CPB circuit is important. The need for a further period of aortic cross-clamping does not preclude a favourable outcome.

Internal defibrillation

- Internal defibrillation using paddles applied directly across the ventricles requires considerably less energy that that used for external defibrillation.
- For biphasic shocks, starting at 5 J optimises for lowest threshold and cumulative energy, whereas 10 or 20 J optimises for more rapid defibrillation and fewer shocks. Monophasic shocks require approximately double these energy levels.

Further reading

1. International Liaison Committee on Resuscitation. 2005 International Consensus on Cardiopulmonary Resuscitation and Emergency Cardiovascular Care Science with Treatment Recommendations. Resuscitation 2005;67:226–8.
2. European Resuscitation Council. European Resuscitation Council guidelines for resuscitation 2005. Resuscitation 2005;67(Suppl 1):S135–70.

Chapter 7
The ethics of resuscitation and end of life decisions

Peter Baskett, Petter Steen and Leo Bossaert

Introduction

Successful resuscitation attempts have brought extended, useful and precious life to many, and happiness and relief to their relatives and loved ones. And yet, there are occasions when resuscitation attempts have merely prolonged suffering and the process of dying. In a few cases resuscitation has resulted in the ultimate tragedy – the patient in a persistent vegetative state. It is to be remembered that resuscitation attempts are unsuccessful in 70–95% of cases and death ultimately is inevitable. All would wish to die with dignity.

A number of ethical considerations are required to ensure that the decisions to attempt or withhold are appropriate and the patients and their loved ones are treated with dignity. These decisions may be influenced by individual, international and local cultural, legal, traditional, religious, social and economic factors. Sometimes the decisions can be made in advance, but often they have to be made in a matter of seconds at the time of the emergency. Therefore, it is important that healthcare providers understand the principles involved before they are put in a situation where a resuscitation decision must be made.

Objectives

This chapter will deal with the following ethical aspects and decisions:

- Advance directives, sometimes known as living wills.
- When not to start resuscitation attempts.
- When to stop resuscitation attempts.

- Decision making by non-physicians.
- When to withdraw treatment in those in a persistent vegetative state following resuscitation.
- Decisions regarding family members or loved ones who wish to be present during resuscitation.
- Decisions regarding research and training on the recently dead.
- The breaking of bad news to relatives and loved ones.
- Staff support.

Principles

The four key principles are beneficence, non-maleficence, justice and autonomy.

Beneficence implies that healthcare providers must provide benefit while balancing benefit and risks. Commonly this will involve attempting resuscitation but on occasion it will mean withholding cardiopulmonary resuscitation. Beneficence may also include responding to the overall needs of the community, such as establishing a programme of public access to defibrillation.

Non-maleficence means doing no harm. Resuscitation should not be attempted in futile cases, nor when it is against the patient's wishes.

Justice implies a duty to spread benefits and risks equally within a society.

Autonomy relates to the patients being able to make informed decisions on their own behalf. This principle has been introduced particularly during the past 30 years, arising from legislature such as the Helsinki Declaration of Human Rights and its subsequent modifications and amendments. Autonomy requires that the patient is adequately informed, competent, free from undue pressure, and that there is consistency in the patient's preferences.

Advance directives

Advance directives are a method of communicating the patient's wishes concerning future care, particularly towards the end of life, and must be expressed while the patient is mentally competent and not under duress. They are likely to specify limitations concerning terminal care, including the withholding of cardiopulmonary resuscitation (CPR).

The term advance directive applies to any expression of patient preferences, including mere dialogue between patient and/or close relatives and loved ones and/or medical or nursing attendants. This may help in assessing the patient's wishes. However, problems can arise. The relative may misinterpret the wishes of the patient, or indeed may have a vested interest in the death (or continued existence) of the patient. Healthcare providers tend to underestimate sick patients' desire to live.

Written directions by the patient, legally administered living wills, or powers of attorney may eliminate some of these problems but are not without limitations. The patient should describe the situation envisaged when life support should be withheld or discontinued as precisely as possible. This may be aided by a medical adviser.

In sudden out-of-hospital cardiac arrest the attendants usually do not know the patient's situation and wishes, and an advance directive is often not readily available. Unless there is a clear advance directive requesting no resuscitation, resuscitation is begun immediately and questions addressed later. There is no ethical difference in stopping the resuscitation attempt that has started if the healthcare providers are later presented with an advance directive limiting care. The family doctor can provide an invaluable link in these situations.

There is considerable international variation in the medical attitude to written advance directives. In some countries the written advanced directive is considered to be legally binding and disobedience is considered to be an assault; in others the advance directive is flagrantly ignored if the doctor does not agree with the contents. However, in recent years there is a growing tendency towards compliance with patient autonomy and a reduction in a patronising attitude by the medical profession.

When to withhold a resuscitation attempt

While patients have a right to refuse treatment, they do not have an automatic right to demand treatment; they cannot insist that resuscitation must be attempted in any circumstance. A doctor is required only to provide treatment that is likely to benefit the patient and is not required to provide treatment that would be futile, although it would be wise to seek a second opinion in making this decision, to ensure that his/her own personal values, or the question of available resources, do not influence the opinion.

The decision to withhold a resuscitation attempt raises a number of ethical and moral questions. What constitutes futility? What exactly is being withheld? Who should decide? Who should be consulted? Who should be informed? Is informed consent required? When should the decision be reviewed? What religious and cultural factors should be taken into consideration?

What constitutes futility?

Futility exists if resuscitation will be of no benefit in terms of prolonging life of acceptable quality. It is problematic that while predictors for non-survival after attempted resuscitation have been published, none have been tested on an independent patient sample with sufficient predictive value, apart from end-stage multi-organ failure with no reversible cause.

Inevitably, judgements will have to be made, and there will be grey areas where subjective opinions are required in patients with heart failure and severe respiratory compromise, asphyxia, major trauma, head injury and neurological disease. The age of the patient may feature in the decision but age, of itself, is a relatively weak predictor of outcome. But age is frequently associated with a prevalence of comorbidity, which does have an influence on prognosis. Most doctors will err on the side of intervention in children for emotional reasons, even though the overall prognosis is often worse in children than in adults. It is therefore important that clinicians understand the factors which influence resuscitation success.

What exactly should be withheld?

Do not attempt resuscitation (DNAR) means that, in the event of cardiac or respiratory arrest, CPR should not be performed – nothing more than that. Other treatment should be continued, especially pain relief and sedation, as required. Ventilation and oxygen therapy, nutrition, antibiotics, fluid and vasopressors, etc. should be continued if they are considered to be contributing to the quality of life. If not, orders not to continue or initiate any such treatments should be specified independently of the DNAR order.

Who should decide not to attempt resuscitation?

This grave decision is usually made by the senior doctor in charge of the patient after appropriate consultations. Decisions by committee are impractical and have not been shown to work, and hospital management personnel lack the training and experience on which to base a judgement. Decisions by legal authorities are fraught with delays and uncertainties and should only be sought if there are irreconcilable differences between the parties involved. In difficult cases, the senior doctor may wish to consult his/her own medical defence society for a legal opinion.

Medical emergency teams, acting in response to concern about a patient's condition from ward staff, can assist in initiating the decision-making process concerning DNAR.

Who should be consulted?

Following the principle of patient autonomy it is prudent, if possible, to ascertain the patient's wishes in regard to a resuscitation attempt. Clearly this must be done in advance, when the patient is able to make an informed choice. In presenting the facts to the patient, the doctor must be as certain as possible of the diagnosis and the prognosis and may seek a second or third medical opinion in this matter. It is vital that the doctor should not allow his/her own life values to distort the discussion – in matters of acceptability of a certain quality of life the patient's opinion should prevail.

It is considered essential for the doctor to have discussions with close relatives and loved ones if at all possible. While they may influence the doctor's decision, it should be made clear to them that the ultimate decision will be that of the doctor. It is unfair and unreasonable to place the burden of decision on the relative.

The doctor would also be wise to discuss the matter with the nursing and junior medical personnel, who are often closer to the patient and more likely to be given personal information. The patient's family doctor may have very close and long-term insight into the patient's wishes and the family relationships based on years of knowledge of the particular situation.

Who should be informed?

Once the decision has been made it must be communicated clearly to all who may be involved, including patient and relatives. The decision and the reasons for it, and a record of who has been involved in the discussions, should be written down – ideally on a special DNAR form that should be placed in a place of prominence in the patient's notes – and recorded in the nursing records. Sadly, there is evidence of a reluctance to commit such decisions in writing by doctors in some centres in some countries.

When to abandon the resuscitation attempt

The vast majority of resuscitation attempts do not succeed and have to be abandoned.

A number of factors will influence the decision to stop the resuscitative effort. These will include the medical history and anticipated prognosis, the period between cardiac arrest and start of CPR, the interval to defibrillation and the period of advanced life support with continuing asystole and no reversible cause.

In many cases, particularly in out-of-hospital cardiac arrest, the underlying cause of arrest may be unknown or merely surmised and the decision is made to start resuscitation while further information is gathered. If it becomes clear that the underlying cause renders the situation to be futile, then resuscitation should be abandoned if the patient remains in asystole with all advanced life support measures in place. Information, such as an advance directive, can also become available, which makes discontinuation of the resuscitation attempt ethically correct.

Resuscitation should be continued as long as ventricular fibrillation persists. It is generally accepted that ongoing asystole for more than 20 min in the absence of a reversible cause, and with all advanced life support measures in place, is grounds for abandoning the resuscitation attempt. There are of course reports of exceptional cases that prove the general rule and each case must be assessed individually.

In out-of-hospital cardiac arrest of cardiac origin, if recovery is going to occur, a return of spontaneous circulation usually takes place on site. Patients with primary cardiac arrest who require ongoing CPR without any return of a pulse during transport to hospital rarely survive neurologically intact, although mechanical CPR offers possibilities in these circumstances.

Many will persist with the resuscitation attempt for longer if the patient is a child. This decision is not generally justified on scientific grounds for the prognosis in children is certainly no better, and probably worse, than in adults. Nevertheless, the decision to persist in the distressing circumstances of the death of a child is quite understandable and the potential enhanced recruitment of cerebral cells in children after an ischaemic insult is an unknown factor to be reckoned with.

When considering abandoning the resuscitation attempt, a factor that may need to be taken into account is the possibility of prolonging CPR and other resuscitative measures to allow organ donation to take place. It is likely that mechanical chest compressions may be valuable in these circumstances. The issue of prolonging treatment with the sole purpose of harvesting organs is debated by ethicists and no consensus exists.

The decision to abandon the resuscitation attempt is made by the team leader, but after consultation with the other team members, who may have valid points to contribute. The final conclusion should be reached taking all facts and views into consideration and dealing sympathetically, but firmly, with any dissenter.

Decision making by non-physicians

Many cases of out-of-hospital cardiac arrest are dealt with by emergency medical technicians or paramedics, who face dilemmas of when to determine if resuscitation is futile and when it should be abandoned. Clearly resuscitation is futile in cases of cardiac arrest with a mortal injury such as decapitation and hemicorporectomy, known prolonged submersion, incineration, rigor mortis, dependent lividity and fetal maceration. In such cases, the non-physician is making a diagnosis of death but is not certifying death (which can only be done by a physician in most countries).

But what of the decision to abandon a resuscitation attempt? Should paramedics, able to provide advanced life support in terms of cardiac monitoring, ventilation with oxygen through a secure airway and appropriate drug administration, be able to declare death after 20 min of asystole in the absence of reversible causes – bearing in mind the very negative results achieved with ongoing CPR during transport? Opinions vary from country to country. It is surely unreasonable to expect trained paramedics to continue with resuscitation in the precise circumstances where it would be abandoned by a doctor. In making this recommendation it is essential that times are recorded very accurately and written guidelines provided.

Similar decisions and a diagnosis of death may have to be made by nurses in nursing homes for the aged and terminally ill without a resident doctor. Hopefully a decision as to the merits of a resuscitation attempt will have been made previously and the matter of DNAR should be addressed for all patients in these establishments.

Mitigating circumstances

Certain circumstances will enhance the chances of recovery without neurological damage. As described elsewhere in these guidelines, this includes hypothermia, etc. Sedative and analgesic drugs obscure the assessment of the level of consciousness in the patient who has a return of spontaneous circulation.

Withdrawal of treatment after a resuscitation attempt

The assessment of the overall prognosis of the neurological status after resuscitation with a return of a spontaneous circulation, but continuing loss of consciousness, is difficult during the first 3 d (see chapter on post-resuscitation care). During that time efforts should be made to ensure that blood chemistry and haematology are restored to normal values. There are no specific clinical signs that can predict outcome in the first few hours after the return of a spontaneous circulation.

It should be noted, however, that the introduction of therapeutic hypothermia after cardiac arrest may have changed the predictive values, and caution should be taken until new predictive values have been established for these patients.

In a very small number of distressing cases, patients regain spontaneous circulation but remain in a long-term persistent vegetative state. The question may arise as to whether such an existence is in the patient's best interest compared to the alternative of dying. If it is found to be the patient's wish not to continue in this state, the question arises as to whether basic treatment such as food and fluids should be withdrawn to terminate life. Generally there is agreement between relatives and the doctors and nurses as to the path to follow. If that agreement means continuing with basic supportive treatment then there is usually no problem. Similarly, if there is general agreement that life should be terminated by withdrawing basic treatment, this can be done with or without the involvement of legal authorities as required in the country. Difficulties may arise if there is a disagreement between the doctors and nurses and the relatives, or between the relatives.

Family presence during resuscitation

The question of permitting close family members to be present during a resuscitation attempt, if they wished to, has been discussed over the past 20 y.

Since then there has been a continuing flow of papers supporting the concept of family members being present during the resuscitation process, if they wish. Many relatives would like to be present during resuscitation attempts, and of those who have had this experience, over 90% would wish to do it again. Most parents would wish to be with their child at this time and would not take kindly to being excluded.

Relatives have considered a number of benefits from being permitted to be present. These include:

- Help in coming to terms with the reality of death and easing the bereavement process.
- Being able to communicate with, and touch, their loved one in their final moments while they were still warm. Many feel that their loved one appreciated their presence at that moment, and this may be quite possible if consciousness returns during effective CPR (as has been recorded especially with mechanical CPR on occasions).
- Feeling that they had been present during the final moments and that they had been a support to their loved one when they needed it.
- Feeling that they had been there to see that everything that could be done was done.

To ensure best experience for the relatives under the circumstances:

- The resuscitation should be seen to be conducted competently under good team leadership with an open and welcoming attitude to the relative.
- The relative should be briefed, in terms that they can understand, before entering and offered continual support during the event by a member of staff trained

in this subject. They should be given to understand that the choice to be present is entirely theirs, and no feelings of guilt should be provoked, whatever their decision.

- They should be made aware of the procedures they are likely to see and the patient's response (e.g. convulsive movements after defibrillation) and the possible invasive techniques such as tracheal intubation and placement of central venous lines. It should be emphasised how important it is that they do not interfere with any procedures and any dangers of doing so should be explained clearly.
- In the majority of cases it will be necessary to explain that the patient has not responded to the resuscitation attempt and that the attempt has to be abandoned. The decision should be made by the team leader involving the members of the team. The relative should not be burdened with this responsibility.
- Finally, there should be an opportunity for the relative to reflect and ask questions about the cause and the process and be given advice about the procedure for registering the death and the support services available.

In the event of an out-of-hospital arrest, the relatives may already be present, and possibly performing basic life support. They should be offered the option to stay and may appreciate the opportunity to help and travel in the ambulance to hospital. If death is pronounced at the scene, the relatives should be offered the help and support of their family doctor or community nurse and bereavement councillor.

For resuscitation staff, both in and out of hospital, it is worth offering training in the matter of relatives being present.

With increasing experience of family presence during resuscitation attempts it is clear that problems rarely, if ever, arise. Ten years ago most would not have countenanced the prospect of relatives being present during resuscitation but a recent survey has shown an increasingly open attitude and appreciation of the autonomy of both patient and relative.

International cultural and social variations still exist, and must be understood and appreciated with sensitivity.

Training and research on the recently dead

Another matter that has raised considerable debate is the ethics, and in some cases the legality, of undertaking training and/or research on the recently dead.

Training

The management of resuscitation and some skills can be taught using scenarios with manikins and modern simulators. But many other skills, needed on a regular basis during resuscitation, can be acquired satisfactorily only through practice on a human subject, dead or alive, even though the design of manikins and simulators improves year by year. These other skills include, for example, central and peripheral venous access, arterial puncture and cannulation, venous cutdown, bag/valve/mask ventilation, tracheal intubation, cricothyrotomy, needle thoracostomy, chest drainage and open chest cardiac massage. Some of these skills may be practised during routine clinical work, mostly involving anaesthesia, and to some lesser degree surgery, but others such as cricothyrotomy, needle thoracostomy and open chest cardiac massage cannot, and are needed only in a life-threatening emergency when it is difficult to justify a teaching exercise. In modern day practice, with practitioners being called increasingly to account and patient autonomy prevailing, it is becoming more and more difficult to obtain permission for student practise of skills in the living. And yet the public expect, and are entitled to, competent practitioners for generation after generation.

So the question arises – is it ethically and morally appropriate to undertake training and practice on the living – or the recently dead?

There is a wide diversity of opinion on this matter. Many, particularly those in, but not limited to, the Islamic nations, find the concept of any skills training and practise on the recently dead completely abhorrent because of an innate respect for the dead body. Others will accept the practice of non-invasive procedures that do not leave a mark, such as tracheal intubation. And some are open and frank enough to accept that any procedure may be learned on the dead body with the justification that the learning of skills is paramount for the well being of future patients. One option is to request informed consent for the procedure from the relative of the deceased. However, only some will obtain permission and many find this very difficult to do in the harrowing circumstances of breaking bad news simultaneously to the recently bereaved. It is advised that healthcare professionals follow local and hospital policies regarding this issue.

Research

There are important ethical issues regarding advancing the practice of resuscitation by performing randomised clinical trials for patients in cardiac arrest who cannot give informed consent to participate in research studies. Over the past decade, legal directives have been introduced into the United States and the European Union that place significant barriers to research in patients during resuscitation without informed consent from the patient or immediate relative. There are data showing that such regulations deter research in resuscitation. It is indeed possible that these directives may in themselves conflict with the basic human right to good medical treatment as set down in the Helsinki Agreement. Research in resuscitation emanating from the United States has fallen dramatically in the last decade, and it appears very likely that the European Union will follow suit. The United States authorities have, to a very limited extent, sought to introduce methods of exemption, but these are still associated with problems and almost insurmountable difficulties.

Research on the recently dead is likely to encounter similar restrictions unless prior permission is granted as part of an advance directive by the patient, or permission can be given there and then by the relative who is next of kin.

Research can still be carried out during post-mortem examination, for instance, to study the traumatic damage arising as a result of using specific methods of chest compressions, but all body parts must be returned to the patient unless specific permission is obtained from relatives to do otherwise.

Breaking bad news and bereavement counselling

Breaking news of the death of a patient to a relative is an unenviable task. It is a moment that the relative will remember forever so it is very important to do it as correctly and sensitively as possible. It also places a considerable stress on the healthcare provider who has this difficult duty. Both may need support in the ensuing hours and days. It is salutatory that the breaking of bad news is seldom taught in medical school or at postgraduate level.

Who should break the bad news to the relative?

Gone are the days when it was acceptable for the patronising senior doctor to delegate the breaking of bad news to his junior assistant. Nowadays, it is generally agreed that it is the duty of the senior doctor or the team leader to talk to the relatives. Nevertheless, it is wise to be accompanied by an experienced nurse who may be a great comfort for the relative (and indeed the doctor).

Where and how should bad news be given?

The environment where bad news is given is vitally important. There should be a room set aside for relatives of the seriously ill that is tastefully and comfortably furnished, with fresh flowers daily, a television and free access to a telephone. There are some basic principles to be followed when breaking bad news that should be adhered to if grave errors are to be avoided and the relative is not to be discomforted. It is essential to know the facts of the case and to make quite sure to whom who you are talking. Telling the wrong relatives is a bad mistake.

Body language is vital – always sit at the same level as the patient – do not stand up when they are sitting. Make sure you are cleanly dressed – wearing bloodstained clothing is not good. Do not give the impression that you are busy and in a hurry. Give the news they are anxious to hear immediately using the words "dead" or "has died" – "I am very sorry to have to tell you that your father/husband/son has died". Do not leave any room for doubt by using such phrases as "passed on" or "left us" or "gone up above".

Going into the complete medical details at this stage is not helpful – wait until they are asked for. Touching may be appropriate, such as holding hands or placing an arm on the shoulder, but people and customs vary and the doctor needs to be aware of these. Do not be ashamed if you shed a tear yourself. Allow time for the news to be assimilated by the relative. Reactions may vary from relief ("I am so glad his suffering is over" or "He went suddenly – that is what he would have wished"), to anger with the patient ("I told him to stop smoking" or "He was too fat to play squash" or " Look at the mess he has left me in"), to self-guilt ("If only I had not argued with him this morning before he left for work" or "Why did I not tell the doctor he had chest pain"), to anger with the medical system ("Why did the ambulance take so long" or "The doctor was far too young and did not know what he was doing"), to uncontrollable wailing and crying and anguish, to complete expressionless catatonia. It may be useful to reassure the family that they did everything correctly such as calling for help and getting to the hospital; however, in the vast majority of cases healthcare providers are unable to restart the heart.

Some time may elapse before conversation can resume and at this stage ask the relative if they have any questions about the medical condition and the treatment given. In the majority of cases the relative will wish to see the body. It is important that the body and bed clothes are clean and all tubes and cannulae are removed, unless these are needed for post-mortem examination. The image of the body will leave an impression on the relative that will last forever. A post-mortem examination may be required and this should be requested with tact and sensitivity, explaining that the procedure will be carried out by a professional pathologist and will help to determine the precise cause of death.

Children

Breaking bad news to children may be perceived to present a special problem but experience seems to indicate that it is better to be quite open and honest with them, so helping to dispel the nightmarish fantasies that children may concoct about death. It is helpful to contact the school so that the teachers and fellow pupils can be prepared to receive the child back into the school environment with support and sensitivity.

Closure

In many cases this will be the relative's first experience of death and help should be offered with the bewildering administration of the official registration of death, funeral arrangements and socio-economic support by the hospital or community social worker. Depending on religious beliefs, the hospital padre or priest may have a vital role to play. Whenever possible, the family physician should be informed immediately by telephone or email with the essential details of the case so that they can give full support to the relatives. A follow-up telephone call to the relative a day or two later from a member of the hospital staff who was involved, enquiring if they can be of any help and with an offer to answer any questions that the relative may have forgotten about at the time, is always appreciated.

Staff debrief

Although many members of staff seem, and often are, little affected by death in the course of their work, this should not be assumed. Their sense of accomplishment and job satisfaction may be adversely affected and there may be feelings of guilt, inadequacy and failure. This may be especially apparent in, but not restricted to, very junior members of staff. A team debrief of the event using positive and constructive critique techniques should be conducted and personal bereavement counselling offered to those with a particular need. How this is done will vary with the individual and will range from an informal chat in the pub or cafe (which seems to deal effectively with many cases) to professional counselling. It should be explained that distress after a death at work may be a normal reaction to an abnormal situation.

Conclusions

Resuscitation has given many a new lease on life to the delight of themselves and their relatives, but has the potential to bring misery to a few. This chapter addresses how that misery can be reduced by not attempting resuscitation in inappropriate circumstances or in patients with a valid advanced directive and when to discontinue the resuscitation attempt in cases of futility or persistent vegetative state.

Ethical issues, such as training and research on the recently dead and the presence of family members during the resuscitation attempt, place further burdens on the medical profession but must be dealt with sympathetically, and with an appreciation of growing patient autonomy and human rights throughout the world.

Finally, the breaking of bad news is one of the most difficult tasks to be faced by the medical and nursing professions. It requires time, training, compassion and understanding.

Further reading

1. International Liaison Committee on Resuscitation. 2005 International Consensus on Cardiopulmonary Resuscitation and Emergency Cardiovascular Care Science with Treatment Recommendations. Resuscitation 2005;67:305–14.
2. European Resuscitation Council. European Resuscitation Council guidelines for resuscitation 2005. Resuscitation 2005;67(Suppl 1):S171–81.

Chapter 8 Principles of training in resuscitation

Peter Baskett, Jerry Nolan, Tony Handley, Jasmeet Soar, Dominique Biarent, David Zideman and Sam Richmond

There are a variety of methods used for training in resuscitation. None are perfect and, in the absence of frequent practise, retention of knowledge and skills is suboptimal. The optimal interval for retraining has not been established, but repeated refresher training at intervals of less than 6 months seems to be needed for most individuals who are not undertaking resuscitation on a regular basis.

Objectives

The objective of training is to equip the learner with the ability to be able to undertake resuscitation in a real clinical situation at the level that they would be expected to perform – be they lay bystander, first responder in the community or the hospital, a healthcare professional working in an acute area, or as a member of the medical emergency or cardiac arrest response team.

Methods

Training should follow the principles of adult education and learning. Generally this will mean an established European Resuscitation Council (ERC) course with small group (4–8) participation using interactive discussion and hands-on practise for skills and clinical scenarios for problem solving and team leadership.

The ratio of instructors:candidates should range from 1:3 to 1:6 depending on the type of course.

Core knowledge should be acquired by candidates before the course by study of the course manual, or an interactive CD, designed for the purpose.

The course should aim to produce an improvement in competence in the learner and there should be a test of core knowledge and an ongoing assessment of practical skills and scenario management.

Sophisticated manikins, simulators and virtual reality techniques may be incorporated into the scenario-based training.

For basic life support, by lay people or first responders, home-based learning using a video or interactive CD with a simple manikin may offer a valuable alternative to traditional instructor-based courses. This method minimises candidate disruption and instructor time and finances. However, the role of the instructor should not be underestimated, and in addition to explaining situations that were unforeseen on the original video or CD, the instructor can act as a role model and provide invaluable enthusiasm and motivation. Group participation has also been demonstrated to enhance the overall learning process.

Ethos

The course should be taught by trained instructors who have undertaken the relevant specific ERC course in teaching and assessment.

Teaching should be conducted by encouragement with constructive feedback on performance, rather than humiliation. The mentor/mentee system is used to enhance feedback and support for the candidate. The aim of the instructors is to enable the candidates to do their best.

Instructors

A tried and tested method has evolved for identifying and training instructors.

1. Identification of Instructor Potentials (IP)

These will be individuals who, in the opinion of the faculty, have demonstrated good competence in the subjects at a Provider Course and, importantly, have shown qualities of leadership and clinical credibility and skills that involve being articulate, supportive and motivated. These individuals will be invited to take part in a Generic Instructor Course (GIC), in the case of Advanced Life Support (ALS), European Paediatric Life Support (EPLS), and the Major Incident Medical Management (MIMMS) courses or specific instructor courses for Basic Life Support/AED or the Immediate Life Support (ILS) courses.

2. The Generic Instructor Course

This is conducted for Instructor Potentials by experienced instructors and an Educator who has undertaken specific training in medical educational practice and the principles of adult learning. Details of this course are given below. There are no formal tests for candidates during the course but assessment is ongoing by the faculty and feedback is given as appropriate.

3. Instructor Candidate stage

Following successful completion of the GIC the individual is designated an Instructor Candidate (IC) and normally will teach on two separate courses under supervision and is given constructive feedback on his/her performance. After experience of two courses the Instructor Candidate normally progresses to Full Instructor status, but occasionally the faculty will decide that a further course is required or, rarely, that the candidate is not suitable to progress to be an instructor.

An appeal can be lodged with the International Director for ERC courses who will make the final decision.

4. Course Director status

Selected individuals may progress to the status of Course Director. They will be selected by their peers and approved by the relevant committee of the National Resuscitation Council or the International Director for ERC courses. Course Directors must be relatively senior individuals with considerable clinical credibility, good judgement, and impeccable powers of assessment and fairness. They will have embraced the educational principles inherent in the GIC.

Normally individuals will have had experience of teaching on at least six courses and will have been appointed Course Co-Director on at least one occasion.

5. Interchange of instructors

Interchange between instructors of different disciplines is possible. For instance, an ALS instructor may proceed directly to be an Instructor Candidate on an EPLS course, provided that he/she has passed the EPLS course and has been identified as an IP, and vice versa. There is no need to repeat the GIC. Similarly, current instructors in the Advanced Trauma Life Support (ATLS) Course of the American College of Surgeons, having been identified as an IP in the relevant Provider Course, may proceed directly to being an IC in ALS or EPLS. Current American Heart Association ACLS or PALS instructors may proceed directly to IC status in the relevant course.

6. Code of Conduct

All instructors must adhere to the Code of Conduct for Instructors, which is set out in the Appendix.

The Basic Life Support (BLS) and Automated External Defibrillator (AED) courses

BLS and AED courses are appropriate for a wide range of providers. These may include clinical and non-clinical healthcare professionals (particularly those who are less likely to be faced with having to manage a cardiac arrest), general practitioners, dentists, medical students, first-aid workers, lifeguards, those with a duty of care for others (such as school teachers and care workers), members of first responder schemes, and members of the general public.

Course format

The aim of these provider courses is to enable each candidate to gain competency in BLS or the use of an AED. Details of appropriate competencies have been published by the ERC

BLS Working Group and may be found on www.erc.edu. Each BLS or AED course lasts approximately half a day and consists of skill demonstrations and hands-on practise, with a minimum number of lectures. The recommended number of instructors to candidates is 1:6, with at least one manikin and one AED for each group of six candidates. Formal assessment is not usually undertaken, but each candidate receives individual feedback on their performance. Those who need a certificate of competency for professional or personal use may be assessed continuously during the course or definitively at the end.

BLS provider, AED provider and BLS/AED instructor manuals, together with certificates, may be purchased from the ERC, or approved alternative manuals, translated if necessary into the local language, may be used.

Introducing courses into a country

Many ERC BLS and AED provider courses are run by, or under the control of, the National Resuscitation Council. The normal procedure for introducing ERC BLS/AED courses into a country is that ERC international instructors visit that country to run a 2 d combined BLS provider, AED provider and BLS/AED instructor course. If there are local instructors (for example, those who have passed an ERC course successfully, or who are ERC ALS instructors), they teach on the course in a ratio of one international instructor to one local instructor, with the Course Director (an international instructor) as an additional person who can support the local instructors. After a successful course the local instructors become full ERC instructors, and the outstanding ones are selected to become instructor trainers. Subsequent courses are normally held in the language of the country concerned, and training materials are translated into that language. The candidates who are on the combined course qualify, hopefully, as ERC BLS/AED instructors. They then need to teach on one or two courses, under the supervision of instructor trainers, before becoming full instructors.

ERC recognised courses

To cater for those countries without a National Resuscitation Council, or where the local council is not able or willing to run courses, or for independent organisations without affiliation to a National Resuscitation Council, 'ERC recognised' courses may be run by training organisations who register with the ERC. They undertake to teach according to ERC guidelines, but do not need to use ERC-qualified instructors. Attendance certificates bearing the ERC logo may be issued, but it is the organisation running the course, rather than the ERC, that is responsible for the quality of the courses.

The Immediate Life Support (ILS) course

The Immediate Life Support (ILS) course is for the majority of healthcare professionals who attend cardiac arrests rarely but have the potential to be first responders or cardiac arrest team members. The course teaches healthcare professionals the skills that are most likely to result in successful resuscitation whilst awaiting the arrival of the resuscitation team. Importantly, ILS also includes a section on preventing cardiac arrest and complements other short courses that focus on managing sick patients in the first 24 h of critical illness when critical care expertise is not immediately available.

There is a large group of potential candidates, including nurses, nursing students, doctors, medical students, dentists, physiotherapists, radiographers and cardiac technicians.

Current ALS instructors and ICs can teach and assess on ILS courses. There is also a pilot project underway to develop specific ILS instructors. There must be at least one instructor for every six candidates, with a maximum of 30 candidates on a course.

Course format

The ILS course is delivered over 1 d and comprises lectures, hands-on skills teaching and cardiac arrest scenario teaching (CASTeach) using manikins. The programme includes a number of options that allow instructors to tailor the course to their candidate group.

Course content

The course covers those skills that are most likely to result in successful resuscitation; causes and prevention of cardiac arrest, starting CPR, basic airway skills and defibrillation (AED or manual). There are options to include the teaching of the laryngeal mask airway and drug treatments during cardiac arrest. There is a cardiac arrest demonstration by the instructors that outlines the first responder role to the candidates followed by the CASTeach station where candidates practise. Candidates should be able to start a resuscitation attempt and continue until more experienced help arrives. Set scenarios are used that are adapted to the workplace and clinical role of the candidate.

Assessment

Candidates are assessed continuously and they must show their competence throughout the ILS course. There are no formal testing stations, removing the threat associated with spot testing at the end of the course. Candidates are sent assessment forms with the precourse materials. The forms indicate clearly how their performance will be measured against predetermined criteria, enabling the candidate to see what is expected and frame their learning around achievement of these outcomes. The following skills are assessed on the ILS course: airway management, basic life support and defibrillation. With a supportive approach, most candidates achieve the course learning outcomes.

Equipment

Most courses are run in hospitals with small groups of candidates (average 12 candidates). The course requires lecture facilities and a skills teaching area for each group of six candidates. There needs to be at least one ALS manikin for every six candidates. The course should be suitable for local needs and, as far as possible, candidates should use the equipment (e.g. defibrillator type) that is available locally.

Course report and results sheet

A course report and the results sheet are compiled by the Course Director and filed with the National Resuscitation Council and the ERC.

The Advanced Life Support course

The target candidates for this course are doctors and senior nurses working in emergency areas of the hospital and those who may be members of the medical emergency or cardiac arrest teams. The course is also suitable for senior paramedics and certain hospital technicians. The ILS course is more suitable for first responder nurses, doctors who rarely encounter cardiac arrest and emergency medical technicians.

Up to 32 candidates can be accommodated on the course with a ratio of at least one instructor for every three candidates. Up to a maximum of 50% of the instructors may be ICs. Groups for teaching should not exceed eight candidates and ideally should be six. Each instructor acts as a mentor for a small group of candidates. The course normally lasts for 2–2.5 d.

Course format

The course format has very few formal lectures (4), and teaching concentrates on hands-on skills, clinically-based scenarios in small groups with emphasis on the team leader approach, and interactive group discussions. Mentor/mentee sessions are included to allow candidates to give and receive feedback. Faculty meetings are held at the beginning of the course and at the end of each day of the course.

Course content

The course content is based on the current ERC guidelines for resuscitation. Candidates are expected to have studied the ALS course manual carefully before the course.

The course aims to train candidates to highlight the causes of cardiac arrest and identify sick patients in danger of deterioration and to manage cardiac arrest and the immediate peri-arrest problems. It is not a course in advanced intensive care or cardiology. Competence in BLS is expected before the candidate enrols for the course.

Emphasis is placed on the techniques of safe defibrillation and ECG interpretation, management of the airway and ventilation, management of peri-arrest rhythms, simple acid–base balance, and special circumstances relating to cardiac arrest. Post-resuscitation care, ethical aspects related to resuscitation and care of the bereaved are included in the course.

Assessment and testing

Each candidate is assessed individually and reviewed at the end of each day by the faculty at their meeting. Feedback is given as required. There is one testing scenario towards the end of the course. There is a multiple choice question paper taken at the end of the course to test core knowledge. Candidates are required to achieve 75% to pass this test.

Course venue and equipment

The course requires four practical rooms, a lecture room, and a faculty room and facilities for lunches and refreshments.

Two digital projectors and computers and four flip charts are needed. The practical rooms should each have an adult ALS manikin with ECG simulator and defibrillator. Four adult airway manikins are required together with the equipment for simple airway care and ventilation, tracheal intubation and placing a supraglottic airway such as the laryngeal mask. Intravenous cannulae, syringes, infusion fluids and simulated drugs make up the list.

Course report and results sheet

A course report and the results sheet are compiled by the Course Director and filed with the National Resuscitation council and the ERC.

The European Paediatric Life Support course

The EPLS course is designed for healthcare workers who are involved in the resuscitation of a newborn, an infant or a child, whether in or out of hospital. The course aims at providing knowledge and skills for the management of the critically ill child during the first hour of illness and to prevent progression to cardiac arrest.

EPLS is not a course in neonatal or paediatric intensive care aimed for advanced providers.

Competence in paediatric basic life support is a prerequisite, although a 90 min refresher course on BLS and relief of foreign body airway obstruction is included.

The EPLS course is suitable for doctors, nurses, emergency medical technicians, paramedics, etc., who have a duty to respond to sick newborns, infants and children in their practice.

Twenty-four candidates can be accommodated on the course with a ratio of at least one instructor for every four candidates. In exceptional circumstances 28 candidates may be accepted with extra instructors. A minimum of 50% of the faculty must have regular experience in neonatal or paediatric practice. Up to a maximum of 50% of the instructors may be ICs. Groups for teaching should not exceed seven candidates and ideally should be five or six. Two instructors act as mentors for a group of five to seven candidates. The course normally lasts for 2–2.5 d.

Course format

The new course format has fewer formal lectures (3). Teaching of knowledge and skills is given in small groups using clinically-based scenarios. The emphasis is on assessment and treatment of the sick child, team working and leadership. Formal mentor/mentee sessions are included to allow candidates to give and receive feedback. Faculty meetings are held at the beginning of the course and at the end of each day of the course. Feedback is also given to ICs.

Course content

The course content follows the current ERC guidelines for neonatal and paediatric resuscitation. The course candidates are expected to have studied the manual before attending the course. A precourse multiple choice questionnaire is sent to candidates, together with the manual, 4–6 weeks before the course. It is collected at the beginning and feedback is given during the course.

The EPLS course is aimed at training candidates to understand the causes and mechanisms of cardiorespiratory arrest in neonates and children, to recognise and treat the critically ill neonate, infant or child and to manage cardiac arrest should it occur.

Skills taught include airway management, bag/valve/mask ventilation, log roll and cervical collar placement, oxygen delivery, an introduction to intubation and vascular access, safe defibrillation, cardioversion and AED use.

Each candidate is assessed individually and reviewed by the faculty. Feedback is given as required. A BLS assessment follows the BLS refresher course and a second scenario-based test at the end of the course emphasises the assessment of the sick child and the core skills. There is a multiple choice question paper taken at the end of the course to test core knowledge. Candidates are required to achieve 74% to pass this test.

Course venue and equipment

The course requires four practical rooms, a lecture room, and a faculty room and facilities for lunches and refreshments.

One digital projector and computer and four flip charts are needed. Paediatric manikins (infant and child for basic and advanced techniques) and adjuncts must be available in each classroom. One defibrillator, one AED and one rhythm simulator device must also be available.

Course report and results sheet

A course report and the results sheet are compiled by the Course Director and filed with the National Resuscitation Council and the ERC.

The Newborn Life Support (NLS) course

This course is designed for health workers likely to be present at the birth of a baby in the course of their job. It aims to give those who may be called upon to start resuscitation at birth the background knowledge and skills to approach the management of the newborn infant during the first 10–20 min in a competent manner. The course is suitable for midwives, nurses and doctors and, like most such courses, works best with candidates from a mixture of specialties.

The 1 d course runs best with 24 candidates, though up to 32 may be permitted. There should be one instructor for every three candidates in addition to the Course Director.

Course format

The NLS manual and a precourse multiple choice questionnaire is sent to each of the candidates 4 weeks before the course. There are two 30 min and two 15 min lectures. The candidates are then divided into four groups and pass through three workstations. There is a demonstration scenario followed by 2 h of scenario teaching in small groups and finally a theoretical and practical assessment by an MCQ and an individual practical airway test. The course concentrates on airway management but also covers chest compression, umbilical venous access and drugs.

Course venue and equipment

The venue requires a lecture room, four practical rooms, a faculty room, and facilities for lunch and refreshments. A digital projector is required in the lecture room and a flip chart or a black/white board in each practical room. Four to six infant BLS and four infant ALS manikins should be available as well as airway adjuncts. Four Resuscitaires, complete with gas cylinders, should also be available.

Course report and results sheet

A course report and results sheet are compiled by the Course Director and lodged with the National Resuscitation Council and the ERC.

The Generic Instructor Course

This course is for candidates who have been recommended as IP emanating from the ALS, EPLS or MIMMS provider courses. There should be a maximum of 24 candidates with a ratio of at least one instructor to three candidates. Instructors must all be full and experienced ERC instructors – not ICs. A key person is the Educator. Groups should not exceed six candidates. The emphasis of the course is on developing instruction skills. Core knowledge of the original provider course is assumed. The course lasts for 2–2.5 d.

Course format

The course format is largely interactive. The Educator plays a key role and leads many of the discussions and feedback. There is one formal lecture on effective teaching and adult learning conducted by the Educator. The remainder of the course is conducted in small group discussions and skill- and scenario-based sessions.

Mentor/mentee sessions are included and there is a faculty meeting at the beginning of the course and at the end of each day.

Course content

The course concentrates on teaching techniques and skills. Candidates are expected to have studied the GIC manual before the course.

The theoretical background of adult learning and effective teaching is covered by the Educator at the beginning of the course. The features of PowerPoint and the flip chart are demonstrated and candidates have an opportunity to present a 5 min lecture and are given personal feedback on their performance. The principle of equipment familiarisation followed by a demonstration by the faculty with subsequent candidate practise is followed in all aspects of the course.

The teaching of skills is based on the four-stage approach. Scenario-based teaching sessions use scenarios from the candidate's original provider course. Emphasis is placed on the role of the instructor and each candidate has the opportunity to adopt the instructor role. The part of constructive feedback is a key element of the instructor role.

On the second day the emphasis moves to assessment and, after demonstrations by the faculty, all candidates are offered the opportunity to act in the instructor assessor role for the assessment of skills and scenario leadership. Further sessions include the conduct of open and closed discussions and the role and qualities of the instructor.

Assessment

Each candidate has ongoing assessment by the faculty throughout the course. Candidates' performances and attitudes are discussed at the daily faculty meetings and feedback given as required. Successful candidates may proceed to the status of IC.

Course venue and equipment

This is as for the original provider course. If the candidates come from a mixed background then a variety of equipment is required.

Course report and results sheet

A course report and results sheet are compiled by the Course Director and the Educator and these are filed with the National Resuscitation Council and the ERC.

The Educator Master Class

This course, normally held annually, is designed for those aspiring to become medical educators for the GIC. Suitable candidates are selected by the faculty and generally must have a background and qualification in medical education or have demonstrated a special commitment to educational practice over a number of years. They should have experience of a provider course and a GIC.

The instructors for the course are experienced Educators. A maximum of 18 candidates can be accommodated with six instructors. The groups should be a maximum of six. The course lasts just under 2 d.

Course format

The course consists mainly of closed discussion groups for the whole course, led by one or two of the instructors, together with breakout small group discussions and problem solving.

Course content

The course covers the theoretical framework for medical educators, assessment and quality control, teaching methodologies, critical appraisal, the role of the mentor, multiprofessional education strategies and continued development of the medical educator.

Assessment

Each candidate has ongoing assessment by the faculty throughout the course and candidates are given feedback as appropriate.

Successful candidates may proceed to the status of Educator candidates where they will be supervised and assessed by an experienced Educator and Course Director until it is decided whether or not they will be suitable Educators to work on their own.

Course venue and equipment

The course venue requires a lecture room and three breakout rooms. A digital projector and three flip charts are needed. No manikins are required.

Course report and results

The Course Director compiles a course report and results sheet after consultation with the faculty and these are conveyed to the National Resuscitation Council and the ERC.

Further reading

1. International Liaison Committee on Resuscitation. 2005 International Consensus on Cardiopulmonary Resuscitation and Emergency Cardiovascular Care Science with Treatment Recommendations. Resuscitation 2005;67:305–14.

2. European Resuscitation Council. The European Resuscitation Council guidelines for resuscitation 2005. Resuscitation 2005;67(Suppl 1):S181–9.

Appendix: Code Of Conduct – European Resuscitation Council (ERC)

The Code of Conduct applies to all who instruct, or otherwise assist, at courses held under the auspices of the ERC.

It is essential that these individuals:

- Fully understand that accreditation, and continuing accreditation, of the individual instructor or assistant is dependent on observing this Code as well as completing the necessary requirements for re-certification.
- Ensure that courses approved by the ERC are run in accordance with the ethos and regulations currently in force using the manuals, slides and other materials to ensure that consistent standards of attitude, knowledge and skills are achieved.
- Behave, at all times, while participating in courses, or social events related to the courses, which are run under the auspices of the ERC, in a responsible manner and observe other applicable professional Codes of Conduct.
- Cooperate with other instructors, educators and administrators (the faculty) and recognise and respect their individual contributions.
- Avoid any abuse of their position and maintain confidentiality about candidates' results and performance.

Index

Notes
The following abbreviations have been used:
ALS – advanced life support
BLS – basic life support
CPR – cardiopulmonary resuscitation
Page numbers suffixed by 'f' signify figures; page numbers suffixed by 't' signify tables; vs indicates a comparison or differential diagnosis.

A

D

E